PRAISE FOR *AGING GRACEFULLY AND STRONG:*
ABCS OF YOUTHFULNESS

Who wouldn't want to age with grace and strength? Dr. Silva has provided us with a wonderful handbook of practical advice and wisdom that can be a guide for anyone who hopes to grow older.

—Stephen Brunton, MD, FAAFP., Adjunct Clinical Professor, Department of Family Medicine, University of North Carolina, Chapel Hill

Melinda Silva's book gives you multiple strategies the everyday woman can use to remain youthful and age with grace and ease. In this book you get a glimpse into Melinda's heart as well as her vast medical expertise. The information she shares is easy to understand and digest. Her strategies are practical and useful for everyone, including the busy working mom.

—Ron Rothenberg, MD, California HealthSpan Institute, A4M Speaker

In *Aging Gracefully and Strong,* Melinda Silva, MD, combines her passion for helping people with her medical experience and knowledge. The result is a book that provides a resource of information, and simple steps to take to improve longevity and overall well-being. The book is written in a conversational style, and while there is a lot of science and research to back up many of the points, it is an interesting read.

—Maria Vazquez Campos, MD, American Academy of Anti-Aging Medicine Fellow, Family Medicine Specialist

Dr. Melinda Silva's book is a blend of the sound medical advice of Christiane Northrup, MD, and the insightful compassion of Elizabeth Gilbert. Vital medical information is combined with personal stories that are captivating and meaningful. This book is for any woman interested in improving the quality of her health as she ages.

—Rachel Goldenhar, Ph.D., Clinical Psychologist, Parenting Expert, Fox 5 "Ask the Moms"

I feel younger and stronger just by looking at Dr. Melinda. She has helped me in a multitude of ways, both personally and professionally, and I know this book will help a multitude of women to feel better about themselves and gain the results they want.

—Mary Burt-Godwin, Blogger at The Mama Mary Show and author of *Dead Dads Club*.

What I admire about Dr. Melinda Silva is her passion for helping to improve her patients' quality of life. She walks the walk when it comes to aging gracefully, and her patients benefit from her 20+ years of clinical experience.

—Chelsea Gladden, Writer, Blogger at Breezymama.com

Thanks to Fox 5 San Diego for leading me and my celebrity/media colleagues to Dr. Melinda Silva. Dr. Silva is the "secret weapon" behind aging gracefully; just ask her patients! Her scientific approach to hormones literally transformed my life—and my skin today is nothing less than fabulous! After the *Queen of Botox* does her "magic" on my skin, I am stopped by strangers who want in on my "secret"...

I battled hormone issues for more than a decade after experiencing a brain hemorrhage (from the birth control pill) which left me comatose for 32 days. I recovered at the age of 27, but my hormones did not! I lost clumps of my thick, long tresses of hair that left bald spots (I was horrified). I started taking progesterone and my hair grew back thicker than ever.

When I hit the age of 42, my hormones crashed—and so did I! Hello, perimenopause! My beautiful hair once again went down the drain, and so did my libido. The hot flashes were just the icing on the cake! Fox 5's Dr. Melinda Silva came to my rescue. She evaluated my symptoms and knew exactly what was missing. She knows what to look for, and most importantly, she really cares about her patients.

—C. Christie Craig, Patient and Publisher

Aging Gracefully

AND STRONG

ABCs FOR *You*THFUL LIVING

MELINDA SILVA, MD

DEDICATION

To my family, who give me unconditional love, endless support, and who are my reason for living.

To my patients, for allowing me to fulfill my purpose in life, and who inspire me to be my best so that I can give my best.

To the youthful spirit in each of us who is searching for optimal health. Here's to the best version of ourselves.

ACKNOWLEDGMENTS

My heart is filled with gratitude to see this book complete, and I am so proud and happy to share it with you.

I am indebted to Bethany Kelly and her team at Courageous Creatives for helping me to get this book in your hands. Thank you for the great effort you all put into completing all aspects of development and production on a very short deadline.

I'd like to thank Michelle Wallach of Youngevity, who lit a fire under me to get my book done so I could present it to the Youngevity ladies at Oprah's *Live Your Best Life* Tour. I appreciate your belief in me and I am so grateful for your friendship and mentorship as a successful entrepreneur. You are a role model of aging gracefully and strong.

Thank you to each one of my patients who trust me with their health and allow me to treat them. You enrich my life, and it is my honor and privilege to take care of you. Each of you has helped me to become a better doctor and I appreciate you allowing me to share your stories.

I am most grateful for my family, for your loving support while I was focused on writing this book. Thanks to my children, who are my moral compass and make me a better person by reminding me of what is most important in life. And to my best friend, lover, and husband—my dear Rafael, thank you for all the sacrifices you make for me and our family. I love you more than you can ever know.

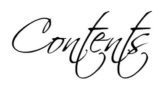

Contents

PREFACE

Many women are surprised when I tell them that it is not necessary to suffer from menopausal or perimenopausal symptoms. Most expect to suffer through this "rite of passage" and endure the emotional and physical symptoms, no matter how difficult.

Has your physician told you that your symptoms are simply the normal signs of aging? Is it normal to suffer and allow your body to slowly shut itself down as you age? What does normal even mean? I say that normal is what YOU say it is. I am a woman and a physician who refused to accept what many others call normal. The aging process does not have to mean sacrificing your quality of life. With this book I want to help you to see how you can become the best version of yourself.

I'm Dr. Melinda Silva. I'm 51 years old and I am on the front lines of reality-changing work with bioidentical hormones and other treatments to create optimal health. When I think of optimal health, I consider the multifaceted dimensions that make up our overall health. Besides the many physical components, there are emotional, psychological, and spiritual ones as well. The combined components determine your overall level of well-being. My focus is not only on length of life but also on quality of life.

I am able to help you because I helped myself. Hormonal changes left me unrecognizable: I was tired but I could not sleep well. I had brain fog and I forgot where I parked my car. I wanted to exercise but I had no stamina. I became snappy and impatient with those I loved. My belly started to get soft and my hair was falling out. I did not enjoy sex as much. The answer my doctor gave me was a prescription for Prozac and birth control pills! In my quest for better health and increased quality of life, I learned how to get my life back safely and effectively with bioidentical hormone therapies and important lifestyle modifications. This book will introduce the tools I used and describe real patient experiences.

I graduated from UC Davis Medical School in 1993 and worked as a Board-Certified Family Medicine doctor until 2010. I completed my fellowship in Regenerative Medicine and now am board certified as a functional medicine doctor focusing on bioidentical hormone and alternative healing therapies. Early in my career, I was medical director of a free clinic for the underserved and worked in a homeless clinic. I have vast clinical experience treating the full spectrum of patients, from newborns to the elderly. The fragility of life at its final stages has deeply impressed me.

People often ask me why I switched from mainstream medicine to functional medicine. Functional medicine focuses on early detection, prevention, and treatment of age-related dysfunctions and diseases. Mainstream conventional medicine, meanwhile, focuses on diagnosing disease and giving medications to treat symptoms. The philosophy and perspective of functional medicine is totally different from conventional medicine. The philosophy of functional medicine is to look for the underlying cause of disease and focus on wellness. It is much more patient-centered than disease-centered. The focus is on personalized medicine with the goal of increasing the quality of life. In functional medicine we understand that every patient is different and that there is biochemical individuality. The treatments we prescribe are specific to each patient.

Functional medicine is based on cutting-edge scientific evidence, using advanced biotechnology. It focuses on the treatment of age-related diseases with treatments such as hormones, stem cell therapeutics, genetic engineering, and genomics.

Another important philosophy of functional medicine is that our bodily functions are interconnected. For example, a nutritional deficiency can cause hormonal disturbances or worsen autoimmune disorders such as arthritis.

It has been so rewarding for me as a physician to be able to take people off of unnecessary medications and treat the underlying cause of their chronic disease. Unfortunately, many women over fifty in the United States who suffer from symptoms of menopause such as headaches and insomnia are treated with pharmaceutical drugs that they may not need. Because mainstream medicine is quick to treat the symptoms without addressing the cause, doctors may offer a prescription for a symptom while ignoring the underlying disease process.

In my previous mainstream medical practice, it was not uncommon for me to see a menopausal patient who suffered from insomnia, headaches, anxiety, and stomach problems. It would also not be uncommon for that woman to be prescribed Ambien for her insomnia, Motrin for her headaches, Prozac for her anxiety, and Prilosec for her abdominal pain. Unfortunately, many such patients would also suffer side effects from the medicines they were taking. What was the solution for the side effects? More medicine! It was not uncommon to see patients regularly taking ten or more meds—most of them unnecessary.

Women have a tendency to put the care of others first and our own care last. It is difficult for us to focus on our own needs when we are also focused on being a good mother, wife, sister, daughter, friend, or employee. Yes, it is normal for our body to experience changes as we age, but we live in an age where we have options that can ameliorate the suffering. We don't have to suffer!

As a physician practicing functional medicine, I carefully consider a woman's symptoms and ask whether they could be a result of hormonal deficiency. Could there be a nutritional deficiency? Could her symptoms be a result of environmental toxins? Could she have a poor response to stress? Could it be the result of neurotransmitter deficiencies or imbalances in the brain? I have many sophisticated tests available to evaluate chemical imbalances, hormonal deficiencies, and toxins that may be affecting bodily function.

I am passionate about educating my patients as to what is happening to their bodies. We feel much more in control when we understand what is going on. That's a big reason why I wrote this book. I want women to have the information and tools they need to be their best health advocate. I want to provide information and tools that every woman can apply to age gracefully and strong. I believe we make great choices for our health when we are educated about our bodies and how they function, and we have information regarding our options.

I wanted to create a handbook on smart, healthy aging. Much of this book is written in a very conversational style. When writing it, I imagined I was talking to a friend or patient. I wanted to include not only information but also practical tips that every woman can use. In addition to education on specifics such as the best diet to prevent dementia or heart disease, I also want you to understand that there are many things you can do to make your mind stronger, to feel more emotionally centered, to feel empowered, even to sleep better! I don't want any woman to believe that she has to feel lousy when approaching midlife. It's simply not true.

I would feel that I have succeeded with this book if someone were to react with an, "Aha! I *knew* there was an answer to my symptoms of hormonal changes, and that the solution doesn't have to involve anything that could increase the chance of breast cancer, heart disease, or stroke."

I want someone to read this book and think, "This would be perfect for my Aunt Mary!" or "…for my mom, who I know is suffering."

As a medical doctor, I would be remiss if I did not stress the importance of proper healthcare and medical supervision. It would not be wise to pick up this book and treat yourself. I would like to see you use this book in conjunction with a competent healthcare provider. I believe the more education someone has about her health and physical functions, the more empowered she is to help herself. I do encourage you to use the information in this book to help you determine your options and to knowledgeably discuss your health with your doctor.

INTRODUCTION

While we can't stop the aging process entirely, we can slow it down. This book gives you many of the tools you'll need to age gracefully and strong.

There is a lot of information in this book on a wide range of topics, and it could seem overwhelming. To best assimilate the information, I recommend focusing on one letter of the alphabet each day. Each chapter ends with an action step, something I recommend you do in order to improve your overall wellness in that area. Please don't just read the chapter—take action. Feel free to use a personal journal in conjunction with the action steps of this book.

This book gives you an opportunity to increase the quality of your life through wellness. If you focus on one letter of the alphabet each day, and follow through with the action steps, within a month you are going to be aware of the skills and changes needed to see significant improvement in your overall health.

Just as aging is a process, implementing changes that positively affect your health is a process. You will experience an evolution of your health, over time.

You may not be able to implement everything the first time you read the book. I recommend you pick up the book again in a couple of months. Like watching a movie for the second time, you'll see and understand new things with each fresh read.

Because of the format I've chosen for this book, there are many instances where there is only space to explain something briefly. I consider it somewhat of an overview of and introduction to the many things I help my patients with. I hope to publish more in the future and go into depth on many of these topics.

To boost the information I'm sharing in this book, I have included resource references and links (which are hyperlinked in the electronic version) to various articles, studies, and papers, so that you can do further reading on your own on any topic you are particularly interested in. This way, you can get a lot more information than what I am able to include in such a brief space. If you have a particular health risk in your family, I recommend that you read the additional material referenced at the end of the chapter on the topic.

Enjoy your journey toward optimal health.

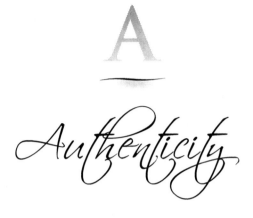

A

Authenticity

"Authenticity is a collection of choices that we have to make every day. It's about the choice to show up and be real. The choice to be honest. The choice to let our true selves be seen."

—Brené Brown, *The Gifts of Imperfection:*
Let Go of Who You Think You're Supposed to Be and Embrace Who You Are

Often people live according to someone else's truth. It might be their husband, their mother, or someone else who they're trying to please. What about you? Do you know what your truth is?

Professionally, we need to follow a path that is meaningful and fulfilling, that rings true with what we really want to do.

Yesterday I had a conversation with a friend of mine who comes from a very strict East Indian background. Long ago, her mother made plans for her life—choosing both the man that she was going to marry and her career. She wanted to be a teacher, but her mother said, "No, you're going to be a doctor." She also said, "You're going to marry this man we have chosen for you." She didn't listen to her mother on the marriage part, but she did become a doctor. She ended up being a pediatrician, because she really wanted to work with kids. So, in a roundabout way, she ended up finding her truth. It wasn't her exact truth of being a teacher, but she was still able to serve children. Unfortunately for her, her parents disowned her because she didn't marry the man they wanted her to marry. And yet she's happy now, because she found her own love, her own truth, and she's a better person for it.

And think about beauty: What is actually beautiful to you? What does being beautiful and feeling beautiful mean to you? Many women go to extreme measures, such as plastic surgery, because they think their body "should" look a certain way. They're forming themselves to fit a certain ideal, usually because it's something that someone else thinks is beautiful, that they may or may not feel comfortable with.

Before you do anything drastic to your body, ask yourself: Is that genuinely what you want? And what is the reason you want to do it? When people don't live according to their truth, when they are not their true selves, they live with a lot of regret. I don't want to live with regret, and I don't want other women to live with regret.

Sometimes women get involved in relationships that are damaging to them, because they're trying to save another person, or help that person, or because there is something about being with a person that makes them feel good. But that person might be toxic in your life, draining you emotionally, affecting you negatively. And any time you have somebody that drains you, you're left without energy for other things in your life. Being authentic with your emotions may mean going down your list of friends and family and pulling away from those who are toxic. Nobody wants to hear that or do that, but sometimes you have to.

When my third son was five years old, he asked me, "Mama, do I have to be friends with everyone?" It was an aha moment for me. What a profound question from a five-year-old. He said, "You told me before, Mama, that if someone's not nice to you, or somebody else, you don't have to be their friend." He went on to tell me how there was a bully at school, and he didn't like how this kid bullied other kids. "I don't want kids to think that I'm a bully, and they might think I am if I'm his friend. So do I have to be his friend?"

I said, "No, you do not. And I'm so happy that you thought about that. But I still want you to be kind to him." And he said,

"Oh, yes, Mama. You always told me to be nice to people, so I'm nice to him, but I just don't want to be his friend." He was already finding his authentic self at five years old.

He helped me realize that I wasn't being authentic in my relationships with certain people. I started looking at my relationships with newfound clarity, asking, "Why are they still in my life?" Or "Why am I friends with them?" In my job as a doctor, I'm always trying to help and save people, and there are people that I really can't save, because they're not ready to make the necessary changes to help themselves. I thought about people in my life who were toxic that I didn't need to have an ongoing relationship with. There was a wave of relief; stress was lifted. And all of a sudden, time was freed up on my calendar.

Becoming authentic often means a departure from things that you normally do. And then when you leave off pursuing things that are not true to the real you, you worry: What are the consequences? What am I going to lose? Well, there is some risk— you might lose a job, or a relationship, or lower your standing in some people's eyes. But what you gain is worth it. When you are true to yourself, to who you really are, to what you really want, then you are free to invest your time and expend your energy on what matters to you. You become far less stressed because you're not wasting precious resources on being something that you're not, for someone else. It takes much less energy to be who you are than who somebody else wants you to be. As the saying goes, "Be yourself; everyone else is already taken."

When you embrace your truth, then you have less stress in your life. One of the tenets of healthy aging is minimizing stress.[1] Something that causes a lot of stress among women in particular is trying to live up to what others want or expect from us, even when it's not what we truly want or care about.

When you are authentically you, you are on the right path to aging gracefully.

ACTION:

SELF-ANALYSIS AND REFLECTION

Are you living your own truth in each of the significant realms of your life? Or are there areas where you are living someone else's truth?

Think about your position regarding physical beauty, relationships, family, religious/spiritual beliefs, and your professional and personal life.

Do you feel fulfilled in your professional career, your home life, and your relationships?

What is beautiful to you? What is your definition of beauty? What does that mean to you?

What does good health mean to you? (For some people, it might mean getting strong enough to run a marathon. For someone else, it might mean not having wrinkles. For others, it might just be about feeling good.)

How can you introduce more authenticity into your life?

NOTES:

1. McEwen, Bruce S. "Physiology and neurobiology of stress and adaptation: central role of the brain." *Physiological reviews* 87, no. 3 (2007): 873–904. **http://physrev.physiology.org/content/87/3/873.short**

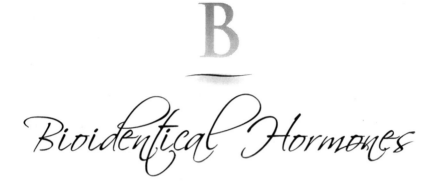

B

Bioidentical Hormones

"When Mama's not happy, nobody's happy."

—Often quoted by my husband, Rafael Silva, MD

When I was 47, I started having hormonal changes that affected the quality of my life. I had issues with sleep, energy, mood, sex, stamina, and weight. I became unrecognizable to my family, and worst of all, to myself. After my fourth baby, at age 40, for the first time I couldn't lose the baby fat, especially around the belly, even with exercise and a good diet. I felt frustrated and knew I needed to get help.

My doctor wanted to put me on Prozac and birth control pills, and I knew that wasn't going to be an option for me. I knew for sure

I did not have a Prozac deficiency! Also, because of my migraine headaches, I had a high risk of stroke if I took birth control pills. There is research showing that women with migraine headaches who take birth control pills, especially after 35 years of age, have up to four times the risk of stroke compared to women with migraines who do not take birth control pills.[1,2]

There had to be another option. Advances in medicine have allowed for heart transplants and even face transplants,[3] but doctors couldn't help me with my hormones and hot flashes? I had to find a solution, even if it meant looking outside of mainstream medicine. Meanwhile, my supportive husband was eager for me to find an answer as well!

While on my quest to find relief for my symptoms and regain my quality of life, I found out about bioidentical hormones, which are hormones with the same molecular structure as those found in the human body.[4]

Synthetic hormones (the ones most women are prescribed) are synthesized from horse's urine, or from chemicals that are not made in the human body. Bioidentical hormones differ in that they are made from natural substances such as yam or soy. The body recognizes the bioidentical hormones as the same chemicals that it produces. The bioidentical hormones imitate nature, replacing what nature has lost. This means that you're not going to have nearly the same kind of side effects or problems as with synthetic hormones.[5]

With my hormonal changes, my hair was thinning and wouldn't grow past my shoulders. With bioidentical hormones, I have thicker, longer hair again. I started sleeping well again. I had more energy. I got my waist back, and I felt sexy again. I got my libido back! Best of all, my mood became pleasant. I was no longer snappy and impatient and I returned to being the nurturing mother that my kids knew, and the loving wife that my husband knew.

I made the sacrifice to leave my comfortable job as a family doctor in an HMO practice to open my private clinic in order to help other women "get their life back." I spent two years in a fellowship dedicated to learning about functional and integrative medicine with a focus on bioidentical hormone therapy. When I was in mainstream medicine, my focus was on disease and illness and treating symptoms with prescription drugs. Now, as a practitioner of integrative medicine, my focus is on wellness. Since I have been a medical doctor for over 20 years, I am now able to bridge the world between mainstream and functional medicine, and focus on prevention of disease and quality of life.

A lot of women go through these hormonal changes and just suffer through them, because they don't think there is a safe alternative. Even I, as a doctor, saw menopause as a rite of passage. Then I realized that I didn't have to live with the negative symptoms associated with it. You don't have to live with uncomfortable and painful symptoms. You can choose to age gracefully and not suffer!

Bioidentical hormones were actually discovered prior to synthetic hormones. Pharmaceutical companies could not patent the bioidenticals because they are naturally occurring substances. (It is unlawful to patent naturally occurring substances such as food, water, etc.) So, instead, mainstream medicine has opted to synthesize estrogen from the urine of a pregnant horse, even though it's much stronger than human estrogen.

Premarin, made from these synthesized hormones, was one of the most profitable drugs in the world until 2002, when the Women's Health Initiative (WHI) study showed that Prempro (combination of Premarin and Provera) increased a woman's risk of breast cancer, stroke, and heart disease (with the Progestin or Provera proving to be the more risky synthetic hormone). The WHI study did not include bioidentical hormones.[6,7]

In 2005, the French E3N study, published in the *International Journal of Cancer*, demonstrated that women on bioidentical hormone replacement had equal or lower risk of breast cancer than women without hormone replacement.[8] The French E3N study also demonstrated that the bioidentical hormone progesterone decreased a woman's risk of stroke as compared to women without any hormone replacement. An important research study from 2013 showed that the administration of bioidentical hormones with appropriate monitoring was safe and effective in reducing menopausal symptoms without causing cardiovascular events, breast cancer, or mammographic abnormalities.[9]

Our hormones manage so many things in our bodies, from head to toe. There are hormone receptors in our brain, our muscles, our bones. Menopause is the drastic reduction of hormone production in a woman's ovaries—mainly estrogen, progesterone, and yes, testosterone.

Testosterone helps women with mental clarity, confidence, motivation, and libido. Testosterone helps women to have lean muscle mass, so it helps them with weight. Testosterone also strengthens bone health. Since women have lower testosterone levels, it is not surprising that women have a much higher risk of osteoporosis compared to men. That is why you see many more women with hip fractures compared to men. Hip fractures are a huge global problem, accounting for many hospitalizations among the elderly and diminished quality of life.[10,11]

Estrogen, progesterone, and testosterone can all be given as bioidentical hormones.

Most women will have suboptimal thyroid function after age 40, which affects weight and metabolism, as well as hair and skin. Thyroid hormones may also be given as a "desiccated thyroid," which contains T4 and T3 (considered the active hormone). Synthetic thyroid hormones in preparations such as levothyroxine only contain T4. Thyroid hormones affect the functioning of the sexual hormones. One of my mentors, a leading educator for anti-aging medicine, described hormones as analogous to the instruments in a symphony. The hormones have to work together in harmony to function optimally.

As a medical doctor, I am well aware that there is a place for mainstream medicine, including prescription drugs. However, I do not want to reflexively give women prescription drugs, especially to combat the symptoms of menopause, when there are safer and more natural treatment options. I do not want the cure to be worse than the disease. My goal now is to look for an underlying cause, implement the proper lifestyle interventions, and to balance hormones. I tell my patients that I think of hormones as being like seeds of a plant. In order for a plant to grow, you need sun, soil, and water. With respect to hormones, the sun, soil, and water are nutrition, sleep, and exercise. Without the proper lifestyle in place, the hormones will not function optimally.

I'd like to share here two letters from my patients, relating their bioidentical hormone experiences:

Patient #1, Jenna T.:

It started slowly.

Around the age of 44 I started to change. My sense of optimism and joy in life began to ebb. My social calendar dwindled away as I refused invitation after invitation with an uncharacteristic sense of disinterest.

The biggest loss was my lifelong passion for the culinary arts. For most of my life I'd been an avid baker and devoted student of every aspect of food and cooking. When I stopped wanting to even read about cooking, I could see that something was deeply out of order, but couldn't put my finger on it.

As I continued to suffer the changes, my confidence and self-esteem began to wane. I was trying to figure out, what was wrong with me? My internal mood became darker and I experienced disproportionate reactivity to life's daily nuisances with stronger and stronger bursts of anger. This was not typical for me!

Lifelong nicknames have been "Sunny," "Smiley," and "Bunny," and I was feeling more like "Grouchy," "Grumpy," and quite often just plain old "Bitchy." In the past I'd experienced a brief episode of depression based on an avalanche of personal losses and I thought maybe my distress was chemical. So I started taking a low dose of Zoloft that was mildly helpful—I was no longer raging about everything—but my joy in living was still missing.

Then more changes. Night sweats, hot flashes, fatigue, and a complete loss of libido kicked in. Well, by then the mystery was solved. My suffering was related to the "change" of menopause. And based mostly on my politics, fears of breast cancer (what woman isn't?), and serious mistrust of pharmaceutical companies, I decided that taking synthetic hormones wasn't a great option. Besides, my medical plan wasn't covering anything at all. So I just continued to suffer. (As did my husband, who had taken to announcing that he would gladly put me out of my misery, but the police would immediately assume he was the number-one suspect.)

The changes continued. I started to gain weight. Twenty pounds. My clothes didn't fit, and no matter how much cardio exercise I did, the scale didn't budge. Then, to my horror, it went up. I weighed more than I'd ever weighed in my life and nothing I did touched it.

While gaining weight was painful and embarrassing and all the other things that weight is not supposed to mean but does, it wasn't the final straw for me.

I stopped sleeping.

All my life I've been a great sleeper. One of those whose head hits the pillow, sound asleep, and then wakes up completely refreshed seven or eight hours later, ready to take on the world. I was a morning person and stayed up all day long and didn't need a long nap every day just to stay awake through dinner. I knew from my training as a psychotherapist that sleep deprivation is considered a form of torture for its power to disturb the human psyche.

My suffering continued.

The light at the end of the tunnel came from my dearest friend, who had started taking bioidentical hormones about six months earlier and reported that her symptoms had abated significantly. Why didn't I try them?

When I stopped sleeping, that was the final straw. I went online and found a reputable physician who offered bioidentical compounds and underwent the testing. After my initial assessment and formulation, I started taking the hormones. Within three weeks, the changes finally started to go my way.

I'm not the type to say this is a miracle cure, but for goodness' sake—I can sleep! My friends have commented that "it's so good to see the real you again." And I have to agree, it's great to BE the real me again. I missed my energy, enthusiasm for life, and most of all, my sense of humor!

My personal experience has been life-altering. I'm 54 and the weight loss remains a challenge, but the hot flashes, night sweats, and extreme irritability are almost completely gone. My libido has returned and I'm laughing again, cooking, enjoying my life, and finding the creative energy to stay engaged with new friends and new projects.

It took me ten years to get through my midlife passage and I only regret not finding relief earlier.

Patient #2:

Dear Dr. Silva,

I wanted to write to you to thank you for saving my wife, Veronica.

For the past three years plus she had been on the couch. She had no energy, not even to eat during the day. Her hair was falling out in clumps. She would sleep for fourteen hours or more every day. She had no strength. She couldn't even take a shower or wash her hair by herself. She was always pale with dull eyes.

I truly was afraid that she would just fade away. She is only 56.

We tried to get my doctor to help her, but the HMO system or his ignorance would not let him treat her in any helpful way. They even referred her to the endocrinologist. He said her thyroid levels were in the normal range.

I went on the internet looking for help. I came upon your website and was encouraged by what I saw. We were both hopeful when we left after our first visit with you. You understood what she had been through and you cared. You weren't cold and clinical. You conservatively explained what we could expect as Veronica started on your treatment plan.

We were amazed and so thankful for her rapid improvement.

After only two months of following your care and using the thyroid and hormones and vitamins that you prescribed, Veronica came back from the dead! She was able to wake up. She had a little energy. She could walk better. The light was coming back in her eyes. Her hair was getting back some shine and wasn't falling out so bad.

Four months later, Veronica is so much better. She sleeps about 9 or 10 hours (always has) and can wake up quickly and can get dressed and brush her own hair. Her strength is almost all back. She has been outside. We even had our first yoga class together. She lasted all 90 minutes!!

I can't thank you enough. I love my wife and look forward to many years with her and you as her doctor and advisor.

Sincerely,

J. H.

The median age for menopause is 51. Symptoms such as fatigue, mood changes, insomnia, skin changes, decreased libido, weight gain, or brain fog can happen as early as 15 years prior to menopause or after a pregnancy. Men can have similar symptoms (also due to hormone changes), and this is referred to as a "midlife crisis." If you're wondering whether you should have your hormones tested, take the hormone quiz below.

ACTION:

THE HORMONE QUIZ

Answer these questions relative to any changes that have taken place in your life and body in the last six months, year, or five years or more.

1. Do you have problems either with falling asleep or staying asleep?

2. Do you feel more tired or have less stamina for exercise?

3. Have you had issues with weight, including gaining weight, especially around the middle?

4. Do you feel overwhelmed or anxious?

5. Do you feel intermittent sadness or depression?

6. Do you feel irritable, angry, or have mood swings?

7. Do you have decreased libido or vaginal dryness?

8. Have you experienced hair loss or hair thinning?

9. Do you have hot flashes or night sweats?

10. Do you have painful periods, or have your periods changed in some way?

11. Do you have drier skin, eyes or hair?

If you answered yes to any of these questions, you may have a hormone imbalance.

The next step is to get your hormones evaluated by a qualified medical doctor. Make an appointment and get an evaluation done soon.

To find a listing of doctors in your area, look here: http://www.bioidenticaldoctors.com/

You can also search for a compounding pharmacy in your area, and request a referral for a reputable bioidentical hormone doctor.[12]

NOTES:

1. Sacco, Simona, Silvia Ricci, Diana Degan, and Antonio Carolei. "Migraine in women: the role of hormones and their impact on vascular diseases." *The Journal of Headache and Pain* 13, no. 3 (2012): 177–189.
http://link.springer.com/article/10.1007/s10194-012-0424-y#page-1

2. Curtis, Kathryn M., Anshu P. Mohllajee, and Herbert B. Peterson. "Use of combined oral contraceptives among women with migraine and nonmigrainous headaches: a systematic review." *Contraception* 73, no. 2 (2006): 189–194.
http://www.contraceptionjournal.org/article/S0010-7824%2805%2900318-5/abstract

3. Barret, Juan P., Joan Gavaldà, Javier Bueno, Xavier Nuvials, Teresa Pont, Nuria Masnou, Maria J. Colomina et al. "Full face transplant: the first case report." *Annals of Surgery* 254, no. 2 (2011): 252–256.
http://journals.lww.com/annalsofsurgery/Abstract/2011/08000/Full_Face_Transplant__The_First_Case_Report.11.aspx

4. Hotze, Steven F., Donald P. Ellsworth. "Point/Counterpoint: The case for bioidentical hormones." *Journal of American Physicians and Surgeons* 13, no. 2 (2008): 43–3,.
http://thefansproject.com/images/fckuploads/File/CaseForBioidentical(1).pdf

5. Holtorf, Kent. "The bioidentical hormone debate." *Postgrad Med* 121, no. 1 (2009): 4–9.
http://www.holtorfmed.com/the-bioidentical-hormone-debate-are-bioidentical-hormones-estradiol-estriol-and-progesterone-safer-or-more-efficacious-than-commonly-used-synthetic-versions-in-hormone-replacement-therapy/

6. Rossouw JE, Anderson GL, Prentice RL et al. "Risks and benefits of estrogen plus progestin in healthy postmenopausal women: principal results from the Women's Health Initiative randomized controlled trial." *JAMA.* 2002 Jul 17;288(3):321–33.
http://www.ncbi.nlm.nih.gov/pubmed/12117397

7. Gurney, Elizabeth P., Margaret J. Nachtigall, Lila E. Nachtigall, and Frederick Naftolin. "The Women's Health Initiative trial and related studies: 10 years later: A clinician's view." *The Journal of steroid biochemistry and molecular biology* 142 (2014): 4-11.
http://www.ncbi.nlm.nih.gov/pubmed/24172877

8. Fournier A, Berrino F, Riboli E, Avenel V, Clavel-Chapelon F. "Breast cancer risk in relation to different types of hormone replacement therapy in the E3N-EPIC cohort." *Int J Cancer* 2005;114:448–54.
http://www.ncbi.nlm.nih.gov/pubmed/15551359

9. Mahmud K. "HRT with Cardiovascular and Breast Cancer Risk Reduction."
J Gen Pract 1:131. doi: 10.4172/2329-9126.1000131
http://esciencecentral.org/journals/hrt-with-cardiovascular-and-breast-
cancer-risk-reduction-2329-9126.1000131.php?aid=20496

10. Kannus, P., J. Parkkari, H. Sievänen, Ari Heinonen, I. Vuori, and M.
Järvinen. "Epidemiology of hip fractures." *Bone* 18, no. 1 (1996): S57–S63.
http://www.thebonejournal.com/article/8756-3282%2895%2900381-9/abstract

11. Cooper, C., G. Campion, and L. J. Melton III. "Hip fractures in the elderly: a
world-wide projection." *Osteoporosis International* 2, no. 6 (1992): 285–289.
http://link.springer.com/article/10.1007/BF01623184#page-1

12. Links to some compounded pharmacies:
http://www.ucprx.com/
http://www.lavitarx.com/
http://www.belmarpharmacy.com/
http://www.medaus.com/
http://centraldrugsrx.com/

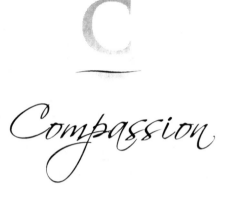

C

Compassion

"Love and compassion are necessities, not luxuries. Without them humanity cannot survive."

—The Dalai Lama

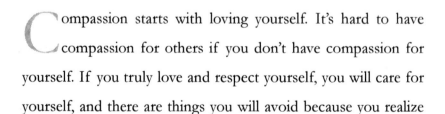

Compassion starts with loving yourself. It's hard to have compassion for others if you don't have compassion for yourself. If you truly love and respect yourself, you will care for yourself, and there are things you will avoid because you realize that they would be harmful to you.

I remember when I had the wonderful opportunity to meditate with the Dalai Lama. I was in a crowded stadium attending an inspirational women's leadership conference. The Dalai Lama's presence was evident and genuine. Even though there were thousands around me, I felt his compassion like a beam of light. He was in his element, and because he was a symbol of love and truth, I felt his compassion as if we were in an intimate setting. I found myself daydreaming about what our world would be like if we had more people sharing true compassion like the Dalai Lama.

As a busy woman and mother of four children, I know firsthand that it's easy to neglect yourself while putting everyone else first. I want you to have self-love so that you have the capacity to love others fully.

I think it's important to have something that you're devoted to in life. For me, that's my family. When I wake up in the morning, I look forward to giving my kids a hug before they go to school, and I love making sure that they're ready for their school day. My day starts with love because it starts with my family. This love and compassion is my fuel.

And then I have compassion in my work, compassion for my patients. I feel privileged that patients trust me with their health. I have a compassion-centered practice, and what that means to me is based on something one of my greatest mentors told me a long time ago—that patients "don't care how much you know until they know how much you care." My practice comes from that core of compassion—my patients know that I care about them. They know that I have a genuine interest in their health, and in each of them as a human being. This helps them feel empowered to take care of themselves. They see me caring about them and offering them the best knowledge I have to help them have a better and healthier life, and I think that energy motivates them to take better care of themselves.

I have had patients tell me that they've been to other doctors that they felt didn't care about them, and they were less motivated to take the medicine that those doctors offered or prescribed. Patients have told me that if they feel the doctor does not really care about them, they are less likely to trust them. And why would you do something that someone asked you to do if you didn't think they cared about you? I think it's important to have genuine care and compassion for the patient you're taking care of, and that's what helps me be a better doctor—and a better person!

I have received many honors and accolades as a teacher and leader in medicine. In my more than 20-year medical career, my most treasured award is "Most Compassionate Physician Award," because it is an honor based on patient recommendations—and received by only one doctor a year at Kaiser Permanente Southern California.

I've had to learn how to have love and compassion for myself. I always loved and cared for other people, but I didn't always love myself. When I first left home and went away to college, I allowed myself to be in an unhealthy, abusive relationship. I was learning how to love myself and still learning about self-respect. I was young and naive and I blamed myself for being in an abusive relationship. I felt as if there must be something wrong with me. It couldn't be the other person; it must be me. I let my boyfriend take advantage of me and of my kindness. He was intimidated by my successful career because he believed that, "A woman's place is in the home."

It was 1981 and we did not have computer laptops, and all our homework and projects were written or typed up one project at a time. So if you made a mistake, you had to white it out or retype it or rewrite it (no such thing as saving and reprinting). UCLA was very competitive, and I recall struggling with a difficult chemistry project. I worked so hard on my final project all night and was ready to turn it in, when my insecure boyfriend tore up my project and threw it at me. All my hard work and dignity disregarded and tossed in my face! Once I learned to have compassion for myself, I had the strength to make the right choices—starting with saying goodbye to that abusive relationship.

No one should ever endure abuse from another, whether it's physical or emotional, especially from someone who is supposed to love you. I consider myself lucky for recognizing my self-worth and knowing that compassion was my key to freedom. I know that many people struggle with hurtful relationships, going from one abusive relationship to another, lacking self-love and self-respect. I feel fortunate that I learned that lesson early in life and never allowed myself to enter another abusive romantic relationship. Self-love cannot survive alongside self-abuse. I am so grateful to now be in a marriage where compassion and respect are at the core of the relationship.

What about compassion as we age? Are there gender differences? Research shows that compassion helps women maintain interpersonal relationships. Also, resilience and significant life events are more likely to facilitate the desire to help others and to be more compassionate.[1]

Some of the compassion practices that I follow, that help me keep the love flowing for myself and others, include things I will cover in more detail within this book: Healthy living with good sleep, good nutrition, and good exercise; doing things that keep my body in the best shape possible. Taking time for myself, quiet time to rejuvenate and regenerate. Respecting myself; refusing to do things that I know will be hurtful to me. Thinking about what makes me happy and actually doing those things. For example, doing yoga for an hour a week. Finding something that I can reward myself with, so I feel that I'm taking care of myself. Doing something that I really enjoy, that is just for me, that feels right to me.

ACTION:

REFLECTION ON LOVE AND COMPASSION

Think about what symbolizes love in your life. Is it your child? Your family? Your pet? Your friends?

Do you give enough attention to that love and relationship?

How can you have more compassion in your life?

How can you love yourself more?

How can you provide more compassion to others?

NOTES:

1. Moore, Raeanne C., Allison R. Kaup, Wesley K. Thompson, Matthew E. Peters, Dilip V. Jeste, Shahrokh Golshan, and Lisa T. Eyler. "From suffering to caring: a model of differences among older adults in levels of compassion." *International Journal of Geriatric Psychiatry* (2014). **http://onlinelibrary.wiley.com/doi/10.1002/gps.4123/abstract**

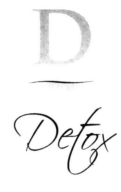

Detox

"*Health is wealth.*"

—Unknown

Our bodies are bombarded with toxins from our environment on a daily basis—from the air that we breathe, the pollution from exhaust fumes, the water bottles we drink from, the grass patch that has been sprayed in the park, the chemicals that our furniture has been treated with, the chemicals we use to clean our house, the lotions we put on our body. These toxins build up in our body and affect our liver and kidneys, causing our body not to function optimally.

To detoxify your body is to remove the toxins that build up in your system over time. Not all detox programs are safe. The products and protocols that I recommend are medical grade and clinically tested. Detoxes should always be done under the supervision of a properly trained clinician. The detox program I choose for my patients consists of clincally tested shakes and pills, coupled with a whole food diet. The detox process gets rid of inflammation and toxins in the body. I've had patients lose inches from around their waist in a matter of days because their abdomen was no longer inflamed or bloated.

Just last week, one of the moms from my daughter's soccer team came to see me for weight loss. Based on her abdominal bloating and fatigue, I recommended she start on my detox program. A week later she approached me, elated with her results. In just five days, she said that she felt her ribs for the first time in years. The abdominal bloating was already clearing, and she was also excited that she could see her C-section scar again, since the fat was no longer overlapping it. The toxins in her body had caused so much inflammation that she had edema and swelling in her arms and trunk area, and detoxifying cleared that out. She sheepishly admitted to sharing the detox with her husband, and I assured her it was fine; he should detox as well. He was also happy to see some quick results—the decreased swelling around his neck was noticeable after just one week. I enjoy treating couples because I know that when people do things together and hold each other accountable, they are always more successful.

If detox can cause such a drastic change on the outside of your body, imagine the transformation that goes on inside your body. I recommend my patients detox at least once a year, maybe twice, depending on how much their bodies are exposed to toxins. Detox will jump-start any weight loss program.

There are different aspects to detox. One significant element is our diet—which should consist of whole food. Some people ask, "What is whole food?" Well, think about the days of hunters and gatherers. Whole food is food that you could hunt or gather. That means fruits, vegetables, legumes, lean meat, fish, and chicken. And as much as possible, buy foods that are free of substances such as hormones that were put in so that the food could be fattened or mass produced.[1]

Another aspect is being cognizant of the chemicals that are present in our everyday environment, which can include parabens in the deodorant that we use, and other chemicals in the creams that we put on our bodies, including the makeup that we put on our faces. Chemicals that we put on our skin will be readily absorbed and can affect our body systemically. Xenoestrogens such as parabens and phthalates, found commonly in cosmetics, can mimic estrogen in your body, causing estrogen dominance symptoms. The xenoestrogens are stored in your fat cells, and accumulation of these hormone mimickers has been linked to increased risk of breast and testicular cancer, obesity, infertility, early onset puberty, diabetes, endometriosis, and miscarriages.[2]

There are alternatives that have fewer or no chemicals that are worth looking into. I am so proud to have helped my dear friend, Michelle Wallach, to develop a mineral makeup (Youngevity Mineral Makeup) that is free of parabens and toxic chemicals.

Also, try to minimize exposure to the chemicals that are spread through the air, pollution from cars, smog, household chemicals, and of course secondhand smoke. Unfortunately, there are many cases of people with lung cancer who never smoked but were exposed to secondhand smoke. There is research to show that when children are exposed to smoke, they have increased risk of asthma and infections, especially ear infections.[3]

Some of these toxins are hormone mimickers, and so can cause disruption of our hormones. I have seen men as young as their 20s with low testosterone levels, which can be caused by the hormones from the meat that they eat, by GMO foods, soy products, or by environmental toxins that they're exposed to.[4] I recall an anxious 23-year-old man who was worried about his girlfriend leaving him because of his decreased libido. His work was very stressful and he was fatigued most of the day, with difficulty sleeping at night. Also, he noticed his hair was thinning and his abdomen was "getting soft." All of his labs were normal, except his testosterone was at 260. The reference range for testosterone in this particular lab test was 230–860. By mainstream medical standards his "labs were within normal limits," but normal for a 90-year-old man!

I was able to treat him and normalize his testosterone (I did not treat him with testosterone because of his age), and now he does not have anxiety, his hair is growing back, he is leaner, is sleeping, and has normal libido. He was an example of how endocrine disruptors or "hormone mimickers" from his environment were wreaking havoc in his body. I was able to balance his hormones with detox, a whole food diet, and HCG (human chorionic gonadotropin). The HCG hormone optimizes a man's testosterone level naturally.

No matter how hard we try to minimize our toxin intake, our body will be exposed to everyday toxins to some degree. This is why it's important to detox our body—especially as we get older.

One reason people have a hard time losing weight is that toxins live in our fat cells. So when our body is full of toxins, our body will hold on to those toxins in our fat; there will be inflammation in those cells, and we are in essence bloated and inflamed.

In the detox program that I do with my patients, we focus on whole foods, and then we include supplements that help to clean out the liver, gut, and kidney. Those are the organs that try to eliminate the toxins that our bodies are exposed to. You can eliminate toxins from your body using these supplements. When you eliminate the toxins, you also end up losing weight because you eliminate the fat cells (via urine and stool) that were holding on to the toxins, and you decrease inflammation in your body.

Another great detox aid is the infrared sauna. There was a study published in the *Journal of Cosmetic and Laser Therapy* that showed that with just 12 weeks of sauna skin therapy using infrared technology, there was a reduction of crow's feet and wrinkles on the face, and also an improvement in overall skin tone. The participants reported clearer and firmer skin. The infrared sauna has many benefits for both anti-aging and detox. Sweating is one of our body's most natural ways to detox and to stay healthy. And the way the infrared sauna works is that it causes a rise in our body's core temperature, which will result in sweat at the cellular level, where the toxins actually live. And for anti-aging, the infrared wavelength stimulates collagen production, which will improve circulation and soften wrinkles. The infrared sauna has been shown to lower blood pressure, which is another way to increase longevity.[5]

You can find more information about makeup, weight loss, and detox products on my website: www.drmelindasilva.com

ACTION:
SUBTRACTING AND ADDING

Think about one harmful thing you can remove from your diet, and one helpful thing you can add to your diet—and go out and get it today, if you can.

NOTES:

1. Whole foods that assist with detoxification:
http://food.allwomenstalk.com/best-foods-for-an-anti-aging-detox

2. Kucińska, M., and M. Murias. "Cosmetics as source of xenoestrogens exposure." *Przeglad lekarski* 70, no. 8 (2012): 647-651.
http://europepmc.org/abstract/MED/24466711

3. Öberg, Mattias, Maritta S. Jaakkola, Alistair Woodward, Armando Peruga, and Annette Prüss-Ustün. "Worldwide burden of disease from exposure to second-hand smoke: a retrospective analysis of data from 192 countries." *The Lancet* 377, no. 9760 (2011): 139–146.
http://www.thelancet.com/journals/lancet/article/PIIS0140-6736(10)61388-8/abstract

4. Özen, Samim, and Sükran Darcan. "Effects of environmental endocrine disruptors on pubertal development." *Journal of Clinical Research in Pediatric Endocrinology* 3, no. 1 (2011): 1.
http://www.ncbi.nlm.nih.gov/pmc/articles/PMC3065309/

5. Russell, B. A., N. Kellett, and L. R. Reilly. "A study to determine the efficacy of combination LED light therapy (633 nm and 830 nm) in facial skin rejuvenation." *Journal of Cosmetic and Laser Therapy* 7, no. 3–4 (2005): 196–200.
http://www.ncbi.nlm.nih.gov/pubmed/16414908

E

Exercise

"Strong is the new sexy."

—Anonymous

You are probably aware of the benefits of exercise in relation to heart health and preventing high blood pressure.[1]

Something that is less widely known is that recent studies have shown that exercise diminishes the risk of dementia. We know that the risk of dementia increases with age, so if we can decrease that risk, that is a step toward aging gracefully and strong.[2,3]

As we age, we lose muscle mass and gain more fat. Physiological changes also cause fat redistribution. Because of that loss of lean muscle, and because the fat tends to collect around the middle, our metabolism slows down, we gain weight easier, and we have less energy. It's important, especially for women, to do weight-bearing exercise as we age. Lifting weights increases our lean muscle mass, which keeps our metabolism active. And regular weight training exercise helps with bone strength and decreases the risk of osteoporosis.[4]

Keep in mind that exercise should be age appropriate for the mature adult. Fitness has always been a way of life for me. During college, I grew tired of aerobics and started Savate (French kickboxing). After many hours of training in Santa Monica and three months in France, I became the first American to earn a Silver Glove (equivalent to a black belt) in Savate. Over time, it became more challenging to keep in shape between the kids' soccer games, Girl Scout events, and my medical practice. It was important for me to be "Fit at 50," and I decided to start CrossFit.

I hurt myself, and I was very upset that I had felt compelled to listen to a trainer 25 years younger than me, who did not really understand my body and its limitations. The trainer was telling me to do the same exercises as my 30-year-old counterparts, and he didn't realize that those were not the right exercises for me. They weren't appropriate for my age and body. My 50-year-old hands suffered from osteoarthritis, and my wrists were weakened with carpal tunnel syndrome. I still have pain in my right wrist, and pain in a tendon that I overstretched. The injuries affected my work life, because I'm right-handed, and I do procedures with my right hand.

Age-appropriate exercise increases our quality of life. It also improves our functionality—meaning that we have fewer injuries. As we get older, by nature we move and exercise less, so our muscles lose some of their conditioning, flexibility, and reflexes. I healed with yoga, Pure Barre, and Pilates. I was able to return to CrossFit, but I was smarter, using the appropriate amount of weight and listening to my body.

Try to establish some kind of daily routine, and look for ways to incorporate exercise into your everyday life and regular activities. For example, take the stairs at work, or do some push-ups or jumping jacks before your workday begins. Better yet, walk during your lunch break, or do some squats if you can't go outside. Avoid the "weekend warrior syndrome," where people try to do too much on the weekend because they're not exercising during the week. This is likely to wear you out, increase your risk of injury, and discourage you from exercising.

It helps if you can find an exercise you enjoy—biking in a park, walking with a friend, playing tennis, etc. Or, find a way to condense your exercise into just 10 to 15 minutes a day that is vigorous enough to make you break a sweat and get your blood flowing and circulation going.

As we get older, delicate knees can be an issue for people, and running or jogging can be damaging to the knees because of the impact. Walking is a great alternative. Swimming is the best exercise for working many muscle groups, and it's difficult to hurt yourself while swimming. Even pregnant women can swim safely. You could do water aerobics, which is great for arthritic joints. Check out your local Y, and sign up for a water aerobics class to try it out. There are many options—but find something.

I tell moms, "You don't have to sit around and watch while your kid plays soccer or baseball or football. You can walk the field while they're practicing. Get some exercise in." What could you do in your daily routine that will add exercise? One of my favorite things to do is squats. Regular squats are responsible for my stronger, leaner legs. I like to do squats first thing in the morning and get my blood circulating fast in little time. Make sure your knees can handle it—any questions about exercise routines should be cleared by your doctor. Since I don't have a lot of time for exercise, I like the local Y. You can exercise while your children are exercising or doing activities as well.

I had a patient who would dance while she was cooking! Instead of just standing or sitting there, waiting for the water to boil, she was doing some dance steps. Think about how you can be more active in your daily life. Maybe that means parking as far away as you can when you go to the grocery store, especially if you know you're not going to exercise that day—at least you have to walk a little bit to get to your destination. Walking is a great exercise, and almost everybody can walk without hurting themselves.

Age-appropriate exercise guidelines:

20–30:

During this decade there are few limitations, and it's a good time to start incorporating fitness as a lifestyle. It's a good time to start weight bearing exercise if you haven't yet, because it is important to building up bone and keeping muscle lean. Aerobic and dynamic exercises such as running, dancing, and martial arts can be a great outlet to reduce stress and the risk of chronic diseases, including cancer. The Centers for Disease Control (CDC) recommend 150 minutes of moderately intense exercise each week, spread over at least two days a week—such as brisk walking or water aerobics or biking on level ground, and muscle strengthening (with weights or resistance bands). If you choose vigorously intense exercise (running, swimming laps, biking with hills), then the recommended minimum is 75 minutes a week.

30–40:

If you were a competitive athlete at a younger age, then signs of wear and tear, especially at the joints, may be evident. If you haven't started a regular workout routine, start slowly, even with 10–15 minutes a day. The hardest minute of an exercise routine is the first minute! You can spread out your 150 minutes or 2.5 hours of moderately intense exercise throughout the week. Start strength training with body weight exercises such as yoga, Pilates, push-ups, squats, and sit-ups. Cross-training is great to improve balance and reduce overuse injuries. It is important at this stage to use different muscle groups than you're accustomed to. For example, if you are a runner, add swimming.

40–50:

Hormone decline and the stress of life can show up as belly fat in this age group. Consider having a hormone evaluation to reduce fat distribution at your core. Cross-training and weight bearing are great to continue. Flexibility and stretching exercises are wonderful to focus on, as they help to preserve a range of motion and prevent falls. Stretching is an important part of any exercise routine, and more important as we age, to maintain flexibility and reduce injury. It's better during this time to use less weight and do more repetitions. If you start having joint limitations, very commonly with knees at this age, listen to your body. "No pain, no gain" is not a healthy mantra at this time. If your body is hurting, then either stop, go slower, or do something different. It's important that you are doing exercises properly, so getting advice from an experienced trainer is essential. Also, it is important to make sure you don't have any health issues limiting you from exercise, so discuss any concerns with your doctor.

50–60:

Core strengthening exercises such as yoga and Pilates are important to keep joints flexible and bones strong. Also, be sure to focus on exercises that will help to strengthen the abdomen and back. Give your body more time to recover if needed. The American Heart Association recommends 30 minutes of aerobic activity five times a week for this age group. Check your hormone levels if you haven't yet, and also check Vitamin D and calcium levels. Optimal amounts of these nutrients are essential for healthy bones.

60+:

Core strengthening continues to be important. Focus on prevention of injury is vital for quality of life, because if you are injured, there may be a longer recuperation time. Keeping your bones strong with proper hormone evaluation and supplementation, combined with proper core exercise, will minimize your risk of osteoporosis and fractures—which are a major health problem in the United States. Research shows that women aged 60+ have five times the risk of death within one year of a hip fracture. Remember to try to keep fitness a lifestyle. Choose dancing instead of watching TV, go hiking, try tai chi at the local park, or whatever motivates you to keep moving.

ACTION:

GET MOVING!

Figure out what exercise you can start doing today—what 15-minute routine could you take up, or what exercise could you incorporate into your daily activities? The ideal might be a combination of both.

Here are a few ideas. These are things that anyone can do, almost anywhere, and require no special equipment:

- Walking.
- Push-ups.
- Planks.
- Squats.
- Lunges.
- Crunches.
- Walk or run up the stairs to your office when you arrive in the morning, or go up and down the stairs for five minutes during lunchtime.
- Walk the halls of the building where you work, or walk around the block a couple of times when you take a break.
- Walk in the park when your child is playing sports.
- Walk or bike to get somewhere whenever you can, rather than always driving or riding in a vehicle.

NOTES:

1. Whelton, Seamus P., Ashley Chin, Xue Xin, and Jiang He. "Effect of aerobic exercise on blood pressure: a meta-analysis of randomized, controlled trials." *Annals of Internal Medicine* 136, no. 7 (2002): 493–503.
http://annals.org/article.aspx?articleid=715201

2. Larson, Eric B., Li Wang, James D. Bowen, Wayne C. McCormick, Linda Teri, Paul Crane, and Walter Kukull. "Exercise is associated with reduced risk for incident dementia among persons 65 years of age and older." *Annals of Internal Medicine* 144, no. 2 (2006): 73–81.
http://annals.org/article.aspx?articleid=719427

3. Ahlskog, J. Eric. "Does vigorous exercise have a neuroprotective effect in Parkinson disease?" *Neurology* 77, no. 3 (2011): 288–294.
http://www.neurology.org/content/77/3/288.short

4. Christianson, Mindy S., and Wen Shen. "Osteoporosis prevention and management: nonpharmacologic and lifestyle options." *Clinical Obstetrics and Gynecology* 56, no. 4 (2013): 703–710.
http://www.ncbi.nlm.nih.gov/pubmed/24047936

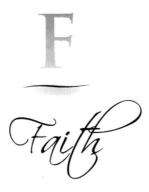

F

Faith

"Faith is taking the first step even when you don't see the whole staircase."

—Martin Luther King, Jr.

I encourage my patients to have faith as an anchor during difficult times. When I say faith, I don't necessarily mean religion, though many people's faith is religion-based—it's based on God, or Christ, or Allah, or a Higher Being—and that faith is their source of strength. I applaud those people. And if you don't have religion, you can have faith in yourself, in a person that you love, in a sense of purpose, in *something* that you believe in. There is scientific research that supports the concept that religious involvement is associated with positive emotions.[1] Whatever your faith, whatever your spirituality, whatever you believe in, having that faith is going to get you through the tough times.

Faith has many definitions and can mean something slightly different to each person. According to one definition, faith is knowing something is there without having any concrete evidence for it. Another definition I've heard is: believing in advance what will only make sense in hindsight.

There are times in our lives when things don't go as we had planned, and when we feel like giving up because it's just too hard to realize our dream or goal. Sometimes we think that the odds are against us. Sometimes people say, "Why even go on? Why even try?" But when you have faith, you have hope that the end result will be right and good, and that's what keeps you going. Faith and spirituality can give people strength when they feel as though they have nothing left to give.

Having such faith in life makes people more successful in achieving their goals. It helps them pick themselves back up after a failure or setback—to learn from the experience and move on. It helps during times of loss.

I thought about Obstetrics as a specialty while I was a third-year medical student delivering babies. It was an exhilarating experience for me to help bring a new life into this world. I will never forget Tatiana. Her mother had been waiting for Tatiana for nine years. Her mother had difficulties with previous pregnancies, and had already had six miscarriages and no live births. Tatiana would be her first baby after many in vitro attempts. The pregnancy was normal, and when it was time, her mother went into labor. When Tatiana was born, she was perfect, except for one thing—she was not breathing. I was horrified. The attending doctor had no answers. He thought perhaps the umbilical cord had choked Tatiana on her way out, robbing her of her life. I could not imagine the pain the mother was feeling. I had a deep ache in the pit of my stomach. The attending doctor tried to console the mother. I prayed that the mother and family would have the strength to cope with this terrible loss.

Ten years later, when I was pregnant with my third baby, I lost my baby at 24 weeks. I felt the pain that Tatiana's mother had felt. I also had the difficult task of explaining the loss to my son, who was eight years old at the time. My oldest had been looking forward to his newest sibling, having said one Christmas that "my little brother was the best gift ever." My son was worried about me, because I had not left my bed for two days. I searched deep to find the words to explain the miscarriage. I said, "Your brother is an angel now and won't be coming home." My oldest son cried and asked, "Why would God want him so soon? It's not fair!" I prayed for strength, trying to comfort my son, and fell asleep in my tears. During this difficult time, faith was the core of my healing process—a process that took some time. "Faith is the strength of life," as Leo Tolstoy said.

Unfortunately, as we get older, the people we love start to pass. The first time that happened to me, it was so difficult, because I didn't understand how profound that loss was going to be in my life, not having that person there. My grandmother, "Inay," was the sweetest woman I knew. I loved her generosity to others. She was only 4'8" but the size of her heart made her like a giant. She used to leave bags of rice and other food on her back porch for complete strangers, because she could not stand the thought of anyone going to bed hungry. I have the faith that I will see my grandmother again in another lifetime, or at least in my own heaven that I have created in my mind, and that faith is comforting. That faith was a tool for coping with pain and loss, and has added meaning to my life.

Spirituality is also healing for people, because it gives a sense of peace and meaning in life, which gives motivation to recover and go on. Among the elderly, prayer is commonly used as a coping strategy to deal with stress and illness, and that has been the subject of several recent studies.[2]

Faith and spirituality are things that we mature in. As we get older, as we get to know ourselves and our spirits more deeply, we can become more authentic in our beliefs, our faith, our spirituality.

I believe in God, and I know that my faith has helped me through difficult times in my life. Yet I don't consider myself religious per se. Having grown up Catholic, I have felt guilty about not going to mass on a regular basis. I have accepted, however, that it is more significant to live a Christian life *every* day than to go to church every Sunday. I try to impress upon my children that the building you pray in is not as significant as that you pray and have faith. I have become more spiritual than religious, and that spirituality has given me a sense of peacefulness. I admire the Buddhists' teachings and have learned so much from their life practices, their mindfulness, their peacefulness. My faith helps me to persevere. I know that the outcome that I want will be there eventually, and my faith keeps me from giving up.

ACTION:

REFLECTION ON SPIRITUALITY

Has there been a time in your life when you had little hope or motivation? What was it that lifted you up and re-energized you spiritually and emotionally during such a time?

What has been your experience with faith and spirituality? (Not necessarily connected to a religion.) Has there been a time in your life when faith helped you through a difficult episode?

What does spirituality mean to you? How do you experience spirituality in your life? How can you tap in to that spirituality more, especially during challenging or trying times?

NOTES:

1. Koenig, Harold G., Lee S. Berk, Noha S. Daher, Michelle J. Pearce, Denise L. Bellinger, Clive J. Robins, Bruce Nelson, Sally F. Shaw, Harvey Jay Cohen, and Michael B. King. "Religious involvement is associated with greater purpose, optimism, generosity and gratitude in persons with major depression and chronic medical illness." *Journal of Psychosomatic Research* (2014). http://www.ncbi.nlm.nih.gov/pubmed/25077855

2. Dunn, Karen S., and Ann L. Horgas. "The prevalence of prayer as a spiritual self-care modality in elders." *Journal of Holistic Nursing* 18, no. 4 (2000): 337–351. http://jhn.sagepub.com/content/18/4/337.abstract

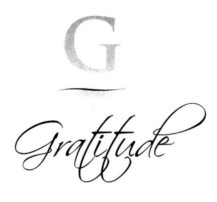

G

Gratitude

"Don't cry because it's over, smile because it happened."

—Dr. Seuss

My daughter asked me once, "Mama, why are you always happy? What makes you happy?" I told her that gratitude is my secret to happiness. I am so grateful for everything in my life, all day, every day. I don't take it for granted that people will be kind or polite, so I am grateful when people are. And because I don't have expectations as I used to, I don't get disappointed as much.

One of my favorite vacations was in Costa Rica. I was impressed that this country in Central America did not have an army. All the kids went to school in uniform, there were no panhandlers, and people were gainfully employed. There was no litter in the streets and it seemed everyone was an ecologist, describing and appreciating all the plants and wildlife. People greeted you with "pura vida," which means pure life. The Costa Ricans also said "pura vida" in response to "gracias" (thank you), instead of saying "de nada" (it's nothing) as in many other Spanish-speaking countries. Every time you showed gratitude by saying thank you, they would return the gratitude by wishing you "pure life." I thought it was very symbolic, in a country which honored its children and environment by respecting both with such care.

My life is overflowing with gratitude, and every day begins with gratitude. I'm thankful that I am breathing, and able to take care of myself and my family. That I'm alert, healthy, and living the life that I want to live. Every day I say "Thank You" to my God for the life I have. And I try to go deeper, and I teach my kids to do the same. I encourage them to really think about the things that they are grateful for, and about *why* they're grateful for them. It's an exercise that makes you even more thankful for things. Think specifically about what impact it has on your life, and also what void there would be without it. What would your life be like without that person, that pet, that thing, that job, that event, that experience?

Recently I spoke with my husband, Rafael, about what we are thankful for in our lives. He shared with me a story of Mrs. Smith, his high school English teacher. Rafael's first language is Spanish, and as a Mexican immigrant, at 12 years old he was immersed into a culture and school without knowing the language. Rafael landed in Mrs. Smith's class, and she was impressed with how well he could read a language that was new to him. He had accelerated his English learning by reading comic books and watching TV. My husband's high school had a 50% attrition rate and was filled with children of migrant farmworkers. Mrs. Smith saw the potential in Rafael and encouraged him to excel and take more challenging classes. Mrs. Smith also noticed that Rafael did not have classes that were preparing him to enter college, so she walked him to the counselor's office and insisted he get on the "college track."

Soon after that, army recruiters knocked on his door, coaxing him to join the service. The recruiters chuckled when Rafael mentioned that he was on the "college track" and wasn't interested in joining the army. The recruiters said they would be back next year, and moved on to the next door in the neighborhood. As a child of migrant farmworkers, he was not expected to aspire to go to college. Rafael realizes the sacrifices his parents made so that he could succeed. His father was recognized at Stanford University for his work as a "bracero," which means seasonal worker or hired hand. He was one of many hired hands working long days in brutal and dehumanizing conditions in the vast agricultural fields in central California. His mother also worked very hard in a flower nursery, to give the family financial stability. Rafael is grateful for his parents' courage and is cognizant that his parents' work ethic has been a source of inspiration for him. Rafael is also grateful to Mrs. Smith for believing in him and empowering him to create a better future for himself. My husband says that "a heart filled with gratitude has no room for hate or fear."

Research has shown that positive emotions, including gratitude, are "extremely important in the relief of stress and in regulation of the neuroendocrine system, protecting us against stress."[1] Related emotions include hope, faith, forgiveness, joy, and compassion. When we are grateful, we improve our perspective on everything in our lives—making the good better and the difficult easier. The result not only improves our mood and emotions, but also our health as a result—since, as we talked about earlier, keeping stress in check is key to aging gracefully.

I think that as we age we can develop increasing gratitude, because we can look back on many experiences and have a longer list of things to be grateful for. Also, we become aware that we have limited time left to appreciate the people we love and the things we look forward to. Even our troubles can make us more grateful; for example, as we experience health challenges we didn't have before, and realize that this is part of getting older, this can make us very grateful for the good health we do have and all the health problems that we could have, but don't.

And gratitude can go beyond something in your mind and feelings. When you share your gratitude by expressing it to others, it makes whatever you're thankful for even more meaningful. It brings it beyond being a thought, into words, and into being a way of life.

ACTION:

KEEP A GRATITUDE JOURNAL

Every day, for one month, write down three things that you are grateful for. At the end of the month, reflect on what has changed in your mind and feelings as a result of keeping the journal.

NOTES:

1. Vaillant, George E. "The neuroendocrine system and stress, emotions, thoughts and feelings." *Mens sana monographs* 9, no. 1 (2011): 113.
http://www.ncbi.nlm.nih.gov/pmc/articles/PMC3115283/

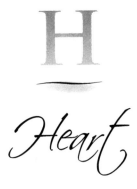

H

Heart

"*What lies behind us and what lies before us are tiny matters compared to what lies within us.*"

—Attributed to Henry S. Haskins

On the day his heart stopped beating, Mike was riding his mountain bike with friends in the hills of South San Diego. The doctors started CPR and shocked the life back into Mike while he lay pulseless and pale in his car. He was immediately taken to the cath lab, where a stent was placed to open up his clogged artery. His left main coronary artery was blocked, and if not treated appropriately could have caused a massive heart attack leading to sudden death. This type of blockage is also referred to as the "widow maker." Mike did not have the typical symptoms of a heart attack. Earlier, while bike riding, Mike had told his friend that he was nauseous and did not feel well. On the way to the ER, Mike stopped breathing until doctors were able to revive him. Mike's only risk factor was that he is a male over 45 years of age. He did not have the classic risk factors like smoking, obesity, or high cholesterol, and he did not have the classic symptoms of heart attack: chest pain, shortness of breath, radiating pain to jaw or neck.

According to the Centers for Disease Control and Prevention, heart disease is the number-one cause of death in the USA.[1] Heart disease is responsible for one in four female deaths in the United States. Even though most women fear breast cancer, more females will die from heart disease than all cancers combined.[2] Although heart disease is sometimes thought of as a "man's disease," around the same number of women and men die each year of heart disease in the United States.

Sometimes heart disease may be silent and not diagnosed until a woman experiences signs or symptoms of a heart attack, heart failure, an arrhythmia, or stroke. While some women have no symptoms, others experience angina (dull, heavy to sharp chest pain or discomfort), pain in the neck/jaw/throat, or pain in the upper abdomen or back. These may occur during rest, begin during physical activity, or be triggered by mental stress.

Race and ethnicity can also affect the level of risk. Nearly 44% of African American men and 48% of African American women have some form of heart disease. African Americans are more likely than any other racial or ethnic group to have high blood pressure and to develop the condition earlier in life. About two in five African American adults have high blood pressure, and unfortunately it is a challenge for many to keep their blood pressure under control.[3]

I recall treating Martha V., a 61-year-old African American woman who was suffering from hypertension, obesity, and uncontrolled diabetes. She arrived at my clinic one day complaining of fatigue and reflux and requested a refill of her reflux medication. I had to convince her to take a cardiac test, and the results were so abnormal that she was sent immediately to the ER. She ended up being admitted to the hospital and having bypass surgery. Unfortunately, because she was obese and had a history of smoking, she had further complications during recovery, with the wound site not healing properly.

There are a few significant things to learn from her story. First of all, it is important to have a relationship with a primary care doctor who knows you. If she had been seen by someone else who did not know her history, she might have just received a refill for the reflux medicine and then suffered a heart attack which she might not have survived. This case can also remind us that the symptoms of heart disease may not be so obvious, and it is important to get the proper evaluation as well as practice preventive measures to decrease the risk of heart disease.

Let's talk about the risk factors and what we can do to prevent heart disease.

High blood pressure, high LDL cholesterol, and smoking are key risk factors for heart disease. About half of Americans (49%) have at least one of these three risk factors.[4]

Several other medical conditions and lifestyle choices can also put people at a higher risk for heart disease, including diabetes, obesity, poor diet, lack of exercise, and excessive alcohol use.

The more risk factors you have, the more chance you have of developing heart disease. Age is one of the greatest risk factors, so as we get older, it becomes more important to be proactive about reducing other risks.

Here are some strategies to help reduce your risk of heart disease:[5]

Know your blood pressure. Having uncontrolled blood pressure can result in heart disease. High blood pressure often has no symptoms and is called the "silent killer," so it is important to have regular blood pressure checks. It is best to check it at a consistent time, mornings being ideal.

Talk to your healthcare provider about whether you should be tested for diabetes. Having uncontrolled diabetes raises your chances of heart disease. If you have diabetes, monitor your blood sugar levels regularly and closely.

Discuss checking your cholesterol and triglycerides with your healthcare provider. The most updated cholesterol testing panel is called VAP, which is a more comprehensive and detailed lipid analysis. LDL particle size is also measured, which can identify people at high risk of cardiovascular disease who are missed in traditional lab testing.[6]

Make healthy food choices. Limiting sodium in your diet can lower your blood pressure. Be sure to eat plenty of fresh fruits and vegetables, which is one of the hallmarks of the Mediterranean diet. Adults should have at least five servings of fruits and vegetables each day. Eat foods low in saturated fat, trans fat, and cholesterol, and high in fiber. Minimize red meat and dairy.

Maintain a healthy weight. Being overweight or obese can increase your risk for heart disease. To determine whether your weight is in a healthy range, healthcare professionals often calculate a number called body mass index (BMI). A healthy BMI is considered between 19 and 25 kg/m^2. BMI greater than 30 kg/m^2 is considered obesity.[7]

Exercise regularly. Regular physical activity will help with lowering cholesterol and blood pressure and help to maintain a healthy weight. The Surgeon General recommends that adults should engage in moderate-intensity activity for at least 150 minutes per week.

Limit alcohol use. Avoid drinking too much alcohol, which can increase your blood pressure. Men should stick to no more than two drinks per day, and women to no more than one daily.

Don't smoke. Cigarette smoking greatly increases your risk for heart disease. If you don't smoke, don't start. If you smoke, quit as soon as possible. For more information about tobacco use and quitting, see CDC's smoking and tobacco use website: www.cdc.gov/tobacco, and www.smokefree.gov.

Take your medicine, and get refills before you run out of medication. If you're taking medication to treat high blood pressure, high cholesterol, or diabetes, follow the instructions carefully. Always ask questions if you don't understand something. If you have side effects, talk with your healthcare team about your options.

Lower your level of stress and find healthy ways to cope with stress.

Stress is very common in our society, and sometimes the importance of managing stress can be overlooked. I recently received a message from the wife of one of my patients, José G., telling me that her husband had suffered a heart attack during their vacation. José G. is a 62-year-old Hispanic male, with a history of obesity and hypertension. He had been very upset that the rental car company did not make the upgrade to his car that he was promised. It was not a big deal to his family, but he was so worked up and stressed that he actually ended up having a heart attack right there at the car rental company. Fortunately, he was treated in a timely manner and survived, but it is a reminder that "stress kills." Also, his risk would have been lower if he was not overweight and his blood pressure was under control.

A valuable tool from the National Heart, Blood, and Lung Institute is a risk calculator (http://cvdrisk.nhlbi.nih.gov/). Any adult can take this short seven-question test online, which gives you the likelihood of having a heart attack in the next ten years.

Based on the results of the test, you can look at your level of risk, and that can help you see if there are things you need to change in your life, and motivate you to get serious about making those changes.

Blood pressure is one of the most common reasons for heart disease, but it's also one of the things that we call modifiable, that we can do something about. Unfortunately, as we age, our blood pressure increases, so it's important to "keep an eye on it." I recommend that you get a blood pressure cuff and check your blood pressure regularly at home. Or at least go to your doctor's office to get it routinely checked, especially if you have risk factors. The goal is to have blood pressure lower than 140/90.

Lifestyle changes—such as losing five pounds, or exercising (even without weight loss)—can bring down blood pressure. It is my clinical experience that balanced hormones will help to normalize your blood pressure. Supplements such as hawthorn can help to reduce your blood pressure naturally.[8] Certain foods that can naturally reduce blood pressure are berries, celery, spinach, beans, bananas, raisins, and dark chocolate.[9,10]

As a member of Youngevity's Scientific Advisory Board, I developed a line of supplements called Cardio to Go that conveniently packages the antioxidants, vitamins, and minerals that promote a healthy cardiovascular system. Supplements are sometimes necessary because we don't get the proper nutrition from our food sources. Remember that whatever vitamins we consume "supplement" our diet, but do not replace a whole food diet.

Please visit my website at www.drmelindasilva.com for more information if interested.

ACTION:

KNOW YOUR "HEART NUMBERS"

You can use the Framingham risk assessment tool: http://cvdrisk.nhlbi.nih.gov/

It's a good idea to have the following numbers checked annually. Schedule an appointment with your doctor if you haven't yet done so this year. A good idea is to have your annual checkup during your birthday month—optimal health is the best present you can give yourself.

· What is your blood pressure?

· What are your HgbA1C and fasting glucose levels? (markers for diabetes)

· What are your lipid panel levels? (cholesterol, LDL, HDL, triglycerides)

NOTES:

1. http://www.cdc.gov/heartdisease/facts.htm

2. http://www.world-heart-federation.org/press/fact-sheets/
cardiovascular-disease-in-women/

3. Go AS, Mozaffarian D, Roger VL, Benjamin EJ, Berry JD, Blaha MJ,
et al. Heart disease and stroke statistics—2014 update: a report from the
American Heart Association. Circulation. 2013
http://circ.ahajournals.org/content/129/3/e28

4. CDC. Million Hearts: strategies to reduce the prevalence
of leading cardiovascular disease risk factors. United States,
2011. MMWR 2011;60(36):1248–51.4
http://www.cdc.gov/mmwr/preview/mmwrhtml/mm6036a4.htm

5. CDC. Vital Signs: avoidable deaths from heart disease, stroke, and
hypertensive disease—United States, 2001–2010. MMWR. 2013;62(35);721–7.
http://www.cdc.gov/mmwr/preview/mmwrhtml/mm6235a4.htm

6. Kulkarni, Krishnaji R. "Cholesterol profile measurement by vertical auto
profile method." *Clinics in laboratory medicine* 26, no. 4 (2006).
http://www.ncbi.nlm.nih.gov/pubmed/17110240

7. http://www.heart.org/HEARTORG/GettingHealthy/WeightManagement/
BodyMassIndex/Body-Mass-Index-In-Adults-BMI-Calculator-for-Adults_
UCM_307849_Article.jsp

8. Wang, Jie, Xingjiang Xiong, and Bo Feng. "Effect of Crataegus usage in
cardiovascular disease prevention: an evidence-based approach." *Evidence-
Based Complementary and Alternative Medicine* 2013 (2013).
http://www.ncbi.nlm.nih.gov/pubmed/24459528

9. http://naturalmedicinejournal.com/journal/2013-04/pilot-study-
evaluate-antihypertensive-effect-celery-extract-mild-moderate

10. http://www.aarp.org/health/medical-research/info-04-2011/6-foods-
fight-high-blood-pressure.html

I

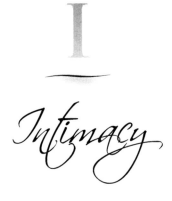

*"The opposite of loneliness is not togetherness,
it's intimacy."*

—Richard Bach

Intimacy grows out of love and attraction for another person. This process of attraction is a dynamic process which is affected by biological mechanisms.[1] There's a spectrum, a continuum, of sensuality and sexuality. We each fall into a different place on that continuum, and it varies too—even just from one day to the next it might vary, especially for women, depending on what time of the month it is. But as a general statement, women are more sensual beings, whereas men are more sexual beings. Women are sensual in that they enjoy the communication or the intimacy aspect most. Not to say men don't, but they enjoy the physical aspect most and lean toward the sexuality side of the spectrum. Intimacy seems to be more important as we get older, I think because it's comforting for us to feel that connection. It provides a sense of stability and security.

All of us want, in the end, to feel connected to others, because humans are social beings. And ideally, as we get older, we learn through experience how to make those connections better. Sometimes intimacy can get easier for women as we grow older, because we're more comfortable in our own skin. We're more self-aware, more confident, more comfortable with who we are, and we feel safer being ourselves. Age will usually give us both wisdom and confidence. We have some advantages in the intimacy department as we age, but we can also face some challenges.

One is that intimacy is very much associated with mood, and so if or when we have mood swings, that affects the quality of our intimate relationships. Feeling cranky or anxious can be a downer. Another issue is energy. One of the most common reasons why women don't want to be intimate with their partner is that they're tired.

Some of the ways I try to help my patients are by helping them with anxiety, depression, or mood disorders, as well as their energy level.

When I talk about intimacy, I am not referring solely to sexual intimacy. I am talking about a connection that starts with trusting yourself, being able to understand what you need. Once you feel comfortable with that, and you trust your own judgment regarding what you need, then it's easier for you to communicate that with others.

When I was younger, it was really important for me to please other people, and I didn't really understand yet that when you're intimate with somebody, you have to trust yourself and feel comfortable with expressing your own desires. If you're always thinking about the other person, then you're not going to be freely communicating your needs and wants, and then that connection may not be so great on an intimate level.

I have had many female patients tell me that when they're intimate with their partner, it's always about their partner. I want them to understand that it should also be about their own needs and pleasure. I tell my patients to get comfortable talking to their partner about what makes them feel good, about what they like, and also about what they don't like. Once you're comfortable doing that, then you will experience more pleasure, and on a different level. But first, you have to know yourself and trust yourself.

Intimacy, in essence, starts with being intimate with yourself. To be able to experience intimacy fully, you have to have a firm idea of who you are, to understand your own identity. Learn to listen to your instinct about what you need. And then you're going to be able to communicate that more freely, more honestly. That will make your relationship that much stronger.

To help women who come into my office with intimacy issues, I check their hormone levels to understand what is happening to them at a physical or biological level. For example, lack of hormones can cause a woman to have vaginal dryness and thinning tissue around vaginal walls. The dryness and thinning tissue can cause pain during sexual relations. The hormones also affect energy level. And then there's the psychological component of our mood. The combination of the physical and emotional parts of intimacy can really affect whether a woman feels fulfilled intimately—meaning both physically and emotionally.

Sadly, there are women who feel that it's okay if they don't get their needs met, because it's expected that they'll put their partner first and meet their partner's needs. Many women I know even feel guilty if they talk about what they would like sexually in a relationship. There are barriers to accepting and understanding themselves, sometimes due to things that happened to them while they were growing up, or relationships where they might have been taken advantage of, or even abused, which can still affect women and intimacy many years after the adverse circumstances happened.

We need to come to terms with the issues on both sides—the biological and the emotional aspects—and be honest with ourselves.

ACTION:

GET INTIMATE

1) Select and buy something to wear that is just for you, that makes you feel sexy.

I like to recommend that women who are facing intimacy challenges buy something that makes you feel sexy. Not something that you think your partner would like you to wear, but something that you like, that you feel good in, that makes you feel confident, and it's just for you! You don't even have to share it with anybody or show it to anybody. It's fun, it's liberating, and it increases your confidence.

2) Think about your physical space and surroundings:

• Is there something you could change in your bedroom to make your space more intimate?

• Are there other places in the home where you could have an intimate encounter?

NOTES:

1. Marazziti, D., and G. B. Cassano. "The neurobiology of attraction." *Journal of Endocrinological Investigation* 26, no. 3; SUPP (2003): 58–60.
http://humanbehaviors.free.fr/References%20-%20Articles/The%20 neurobiology%20of%20attraction%20-%20SCAN.pdf

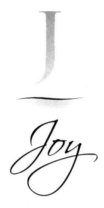

J

Joy

"A joyful heart is the normal result of a heart burning with love. She gives most who gives with joy."

—Mother Teresa, *In the Heart of the World: Thoughts, Stories and Prayers*

When I think about joy, what it means to me is the pursuit of happiness. I've met a lot of people who, when I asked them, "What's your goal in life?" they would say, "To be happy." When I think about that, what does that really mean? Because it's hard to objectify, it's hard to quantify.

I ask myself, "What does joy mean for me, especially as I'm getting older? What makes me happy?" I could tell you the moments in life that I've been happiest, and those moments have always included people that I love—especially family and close friends. They're also times when I felt the most comfortable with myself. Times when I knew I had made the right decision. Times when I knew I did the right thing, even if no one else agreed.

Another thing that is one of my secrets to being happy, and I try to teach my kids this, is to not expect anything from anyone. When you think about the times in your life when you have been unhappy, or when you felt let down, it's usually when you expected something to go a certain way, or expected someone to do something, and it didn't happen. So I figured out—later in life, mind you—that if I didn't have those expectations of anyone else, and the only person that I held accountable was myself, then I wouldn't be disappointed. And I could usually say that I was happy.

I try to teach my kids that if you do something nice for someone, you do it just to be nice. If you expect them to do something back, and they don't, that's when you get disappointed. And then that's just going to be your own fault. So, what happens when someone is nice back to you? Then you're really happy! Because you didn't expect it.

One of the things that gives me joy is being able to eat the food that I like. I'm Filipina, and in my culture we celebrate life with food, as do many other cultures. I'm a foodie, and I have favorite comfort foods. To be able to cook a good meal, and eat with my family, is a source of happiness. Dinnertime is sacred for us. We try to eat together whenever possible, either at home, or we go out somewhere nice to celebrate an event—some place where the food is plentiful and tasty. I usually have room for sweets, in moderation of course.

Also, being active makes me happy. I like music, dancing, and moving in nature. It makes me happy to hike in a beautiful place, to walk by a creek, to see the beauty of what's around me, to marvel at how beautiful our world is. If I have music playing in my ears it's even better, because music also brings me joy. I grew up playing the piano, so sometimes when I would feel sad I would want to play a piece of music, and that would make me happy.

Another joy in my life is taking vacation with my family—being in Cancun, feeling the sand between my toes, being near and in the water. The sand in Cancun is very special. No matter how hot it is outside, the sand stays cool, so you can sink your toes into the sand comfortably.

Really, what gives me the most joy in my life are my four kids and my husband—they help me to understand what joy is. We are blessed to have each other.

I had the pleasure of speaking in front of our local community's Optimist Club. The members were all retired, over 65 years old, and the joy in the room was palpable. They had all made a conscious decision to focus on optimism despite their health challenges and joint pain. Bill T. was thrilled that his lower back pain and knee pain were better after testosterone treatment. He is 90 years old and he is so thankful to be more mobile and enjoy swimming again, something that gave him joy. He told me, "I am so grateful that you gave me my strength back. I am so happy that you are taking care of me. No one has ever taken care of me the way you have. What will I do if you can't take care of me?" I smiled and reassured him, "You are 90, I am 50; don't worry, I will be here to take care of you."

In relation to aging gracefully, I think we need to be aware of the risks of becoming cynical or bitter as we get older. Life might not have gone as we had planned, but we have to remember to tap into our joy. Optimism, having a positive outlook, even when times are tough, or when things may not be going our way, keeps joy alive.

According to research that was cited in the *Journal of Personality and Social Psychology*, optimism can stimulate your immune system and reduce stress.[1] Another study indicated that love and pleasure are capable of stimulating health and well-being in several ways.[2]

Joy is beneficial to our minds and bodies.

ACTION:

BRING MORE JOY INTO YOUR LIFE!

Pick one of the following 10 ideas, and plan to do something within the next 48 hours that brings you joy. Or, create your own list of things that bring you joy.

- Hug a child or a pet. Or hold a baby.

- Turn on your favorite song or type of music and dance.

- Take a walk in nature. Find a park, beach, forest, or somewhere near you that is beautiful.

- Do something creative. Paint. Sculpt. Sing. Sew. Craft.

- Bake or buy something delicious, and then savor every bite. And if you feel inclined, share it with someone.

- Call a friend or a loved one that you haven't talked to in a while. Call, don't text.

- Jump in the pool, take a bath, or splash in water.[3]

- Take a break with a cup of coffee or your favorite beverage and a good book.

- Enjoy a good laugh! Watch funny YouTube clips or go to a local comedy club.

- Treat yourself to a massage, manicure/pedicure, or a trip to the hair salon.

NOTES:

1. Segerstrom, Suzanne C., Shelley E. Taylor, Margaret E. Kemeny, and John L. Fahey. "Optimism is associated with mood, coping, and immune change in response to stress." *Journal of Personality and Social Psychology* 74, no. 6 (1998): 1646.
http://www.uic.edu/classes/psych/Health/Readings/Segerstrom,%20 optimism,%20mood,%20immune%20status,%20JPSP,%201998.pdf

2. Esch, Tobias, and George B. Stefano. "Love promotes health." *Neuroendocrinology Letters* 26, no. 3 (2005): 264–268.
http://www.nel.edu/pdf_/26_3/260305A13_15990734_Esch--Stefano_.pdf

3. Article regarding the calming effect of water:
http://www.washingtonpost.com/national/health-science/
blue-mind-explores-the-calming-effect-that-water-has-on-
people/2014/07/28/471d7a5a-11bb-11e4-9285-4243a40ddc97_story.html

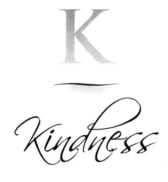

K

Kindness

"Be kind, for everyone you meet is fighting a hard battle."

—Attributed to Ian MacLaren

It was 1982 and I was a sophomore at UCLA. I remember being impressed by the huge corded phone in the shiny Mercedes. The gentleman in the car, an acquaintance of my roommate, was very kind. He talked about how he had traveled the world and met many people, and had learned to show kindness and love to everyone with the same kind of love he has for his own family. It was a novel concept to me—"to love everyone like your own family"—and I wondered how someone could have that much love in their heart. I wondered how someone could consistently show as much kindness toward strangers as they do their family or someone they love. I admired his belief that each life is precious and no one's life is more important than another's.

Kindness has always been a source of inspiration for me. I'm talking about being kind to someone, generous, caring, just because you want to be kind—and not expecting anything in return. Paying it forward. As stated by the Dalai Lama, "Be kind whenever possible. It is always possible." Try something: The next time you go to the grocery store, smile at people and see how many people smile back. Let someone go in front of you in line. Say "thank you" to the cashier. Then reflect on how it made you feel, and on how the people you showed kindness to reacted. See how contagious kindness can be. I know the catchphrase is to practice "random acts of kindness." I say make it more *intentional* and practice "*daily* acts of kindness."

One aspect of kindness is service and volunteering. I started volunteering when I was 13 years old, working for a San Diego community organization called Social Advocates for Youth. My first job was helping the youth in my community be productive by convincing employers to hire them. It's difficult to employ teenagers, because they don't have experience. I was a kid myself, but I would help the other kids with things like interviewing skills and finding summer jobs—trying to match people up with jobs that suited their skills, strengths, and interests. Helping other people to be productive, seeing how rewarding it was for these kids to earn money and make a living for themselves, was very rewarding for me as well. I was fortunate to learn early the importance of being a productive member of the community.

Ever since then, community work has been an important part of my résumé. In my second year at the Family Residency Program at Long Beach, I piloted a program at a nearby underserved high school called "The Doc Is In." The teenagers at this particular high school had a reputation for vandalism and getting into trouble after school. I created the program because I wanted the teenagers to have positive role models—adults who they knew cared about them and who could be mentors to help them make better choices. We did not have traditional didactic classroom instruction. We played games, did role play, and had Q&A sessions where we passed around a hat for written questions, so that the kids could ask any question they wanted, anonymously. I did not fully realize the impact of this program until the following year. On one busy day at the clinic, just like any other, I met a patient who thanked me for having helped him to stop smoking. He said he was sure that quitting smoking had saved his life and he couldn't have done it without me. I was slightly perplexed, because it was the first time I had met this nice middle-aged Caucasian gentleman. He proceeded to explain that his son, Jack, was in one of the classes I had mentored in "The Doc Is In" program. I had convinced Jack to never start smoking, and this teen understood the importance of not smoking to prevent heart disease and other disabilities. Jack bugged his father and didn't give up until his father quit smoking. I saw so clearly that you can never know the full impact of your kindness and how it can affect an entire community.

I have done a lot of volunteering over the years and I truly believe that "the more you give, the more you get." After raising three boys, I was thrilled to finally have a daughter. As a Girl Scout troop leader for the past five years, I have 16 girls. Working with them can be joyful, chaotic, rewarding, and challenging—all at the same time! I really want these girls to have a positive role model; I want to show them that they can be self-sufficient and at the same time show kindness to others and care for others.

My Girl Scout troop is based on service, and I have the girls figure out what kind of volunteering they want to do. Last Christmas, instead of giving gifts to each other and having a gift exchange, I had the girls go to the dollar store and each put together a gift box for an orphan. The boxes were going to underserved orphans in the nearby border town of Tijuana, Mexico. We packaged a few things the children would need—like mittens and toothpaste and socks—as well as a few toys in each box. For some of these orphans, this would be the first gift that they ever received.

It was beautiful to see the looks on the girls' faces when they were shopping for someone other than themselves or their friends.

There was such a satisfaction as a result of giving to someone else, someone they didn't even know. Practicing unselfish kindness had a very positive effect on them.

I believe that we each have a connection to everyone else—that we are *all* connected as one. Kindness honors that connection. The energy of good sets a tone of warmth and a welcoming environment. It helps you make the right choices, to do the things that make the world a better place. An ancient Chinese proverb reads: "An invisible red thread connects those who are destined to meet regardless of time, place, or circumstance. The thread may stretch or tangle, but it will never break." It may not be evident until later why our paths crossed. What is important is that we have the ability to change the energy of our world with the kindness we share with others.

We should be kind not only to people we know and love, but to strangers; as well as to pets, animals, and Mother Earth. Living in a spirit of kindness makes us cognizant of how we treat each other, as well as our environment, remembering that we have only a finite source of energy and resources. That causes us to be saving, not wasteful—to take only what we need, to recycle and reuse. Make sure the plastic gets into the right bin. Instead of throwing gently used clothes in the garbage, donate them so they can be used by someone else. Turn off the tap while you're brushing your teeth instead of letting the water run.

Another part of kindness is being polite. Not everyone has the time or means to do volunteer service, but we can all be courteous to those around us. I am a young baby boomer, and in this generation we learned to say please and thank you, and keep the door open for the person behind us. We look at the person we're speaking to and don't text while we're having dinner. We are respectful to our elders.

I think it's important for children to learn about kindness through volunteering. I ask my own children to "think of something that you like to do, and then think of a group of people that you can affect in a positive way." My oldest son, currently at UCLA, is a wonderful piano player and loves music. So he decided to go into a hospital, to the children's ward, with his keyboard—especially to see the preadolescent children who might not get as many visitors. The nurses loved his visits, because his joyous music would fill the hospital ward and make the children smile. The kids anxiously awaited their turn, as he would give a private lesson to each child. He would interact, he would connect, and he would communicate with the kids, and he was doing it based on something he enjoyed, something he loved. It was his way of giving, and it had a powerful effect on the kids.

I have been impressed with the spontaneous kindnesses that have been shown to me throughout my life. I recall backpacking in Amsterdam after graduating from college. I had been with friends in France, but decided to do some traveling on my own. I landed in Amsterdam and found myself on a walking tour. I had never seen so many blonde-haired and blue-eyed people in my life. I received a lot of compliments for my "unique" brown eyes, which was strange to me, since I thought of my eyes as very common and plain-looking. A gentleman approached me and asked me if I wanted to stay with his family, instead of in the overcrowded youth hostel. I hesitated for a moment, but I trusted the sincerity and kindness in his eyes. He had a lovely wife and two daughters, and the next day we even took a traditional Dutch family picture—all of us with wooden shoes and pointy hats! I asked him what had compelled him to invite a stranger to his home. He said that he hoped that his daughters would benefit from the kindness of strangers, and he wanted to extend that kindness to me.

I recently found a very interesting article that showed how practicing kindness can actually extend longevity. Aging occurs when the ends of DNA chromosomes, called telomeres, are shortened with time (specifically with cell division). Each time the cell divides, the telomeres shorten until the cell stops dividing. At that point, the cell becomes inactive or dies. Certain lifestyle behaviors that decrease stress are connected with longer telomeres. The article showed how focusing on the well-being of others, volunteering, and caregiving, help to keep telomeres longer. Longer telomeres have been associated with longevity and shorter telomeres have been associated with accelerated aging.[1]

In this study, they had people do Loving-Kindness Meditation (LKM), which is a practice derived from the Buddhist tradition focusing on unselfish kindness and warmth toward all people. The researchers collected blood samples from people who practiced this Loving-Kindness Meditation and compared it with samples from people who didn't, and the people who practiced kindness had longer telomeres. What that meant was that their aging process was slowing down. I found that remarkable. And interestingly, the researchers showed that the effect was stronger in women.

During my tenure as Mrs. Philippines/Tourism San Diego, I visited orphanages in the Philippines with my four children. Watching the connections made between my children and the orphans is one of my favorite memories. It was beautiful to witness my children discover that the connection of love and kindness they shared with the orphans was more important to the orphans than the toys and money we brought. To use Mother Teresa's wise words: "There can be no great acts, only small acts of great love." Whenever you have the choice, choose kindness. And remember that when you're kind to others you're also being kind to yourself—and helping yourself age gracefully.

ACTION:

WHAT CAN YOU DO?

Think about a spontaneous act of kindness that you could show a stranger while running your next errand. (Then journal about what you did and how it made you feel.)

Think of something kind and spontaneous that you can do today for someone you love.

Here are three ideas to get you started:

* Write a note and put it in your child's, spouse's, or friend's lunch bag, purse, or briefcase.

* Leave a note on the mirror for your loved one to find.

* Do something for your loved one that you know they really don't like doing. (For example, washing their car or filling their gas tank.)

NOTES:

1. Hoge, Elizabeth A., Maxine M. Chen, Esther Orr, Christina A. Metcalf, Laura E. Fischer, Mark H. Pollack, Immaculata DeVivo, and Naomi M. Simon. "Loving-Kindness Meditation practice associated with longer telomeres in women." *Brain, Behavior, and Immunity* 32 (2013): 159–163. http://www.sciencedirect.com/science/article/pii/S0889159113001736

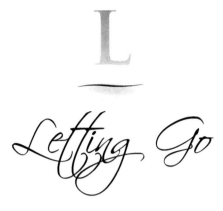

L

Letting Go

"As we grow older and wiser, we begin to realize
what we need and what we need to leave behind.
Sometimes walking away is a step forward."

—Marc Chernoff

There are many aspects of "letting go" and there are
times in each of our lives when it is time to let go of
something. One way is by letting go of emotional and physical
limitations we have allowed to be placed on ourselves. Another
is letting go of perfection and control. There are preconceived
notions, stereotypes, and biases that we need to let go of in
order to progress or evolve. Sometimes it's material possessions
and clutter.

When I think about letting go, I think about acceptance—accepting something for what it is, and letting go of a preconceived notion or bias about it. Working with what you have, taking action, despite things being imperfect. I call that "perfecting imperfection," or as a friend once put it, "taking imperfect action." Sometimes perfectionism actually prevents people from succeeding or reaching their goal—because things may never be good enough to move forward. Holding on to unrealistic ideals can keep you from even trying or starting something. One of the reasons people procrastinate is because they have a perfectionistic attitude, and it's hard for them to even get going on their goal, because circumstances are just never right.

In one study, researchers showed the relationship between stressful life events and depression, when combined with perfectionistic attitudes.[1] The study showed that there is a strong correlation between a perfectionistic attitude and stress and depression. And as we know, stress can accelerate the aging process and negatively affect longevity.

Speaking of stress, something that we often need to let go of is clutter—having a lot of things around, things which once caught our fancy or interest, but that we no longer use or never really used. Maybe it's something that has some sentimental value. A lot of little things add up to a mountain of clutter, and having clutter around us can affect us emotionally—it "obfuscates internal clarity," as one study put it.[2] And there is a connection between hoarding symptoms and stress.[3]

I grew up as a Navy brat, and we moved every couple of years, so I grew to be very sentimental. I was always the new kid on the block and I was always having to start all over with making friends, so when I made a friend, that meant a lot to me. When those friendships would end, either because we moved or for other reasons, it was difficult.

I have a memory of one close friend who I loved like a sister. We shared many things in common, including being colleagues in medicine. We shared many happy times and would laugh together often, sometimes to tears. We shared our dreams and fears and knew each other's deepest wishes. Then one day she said she did not want to be my friend anymore. She said it was because I was "too happy and fortunate in life." There was one big thing that we didn't have in common—I was as optimistic as she was pessimistic. The same thing could happen to us, and I would try to see the "good" from the experience, whereas she would point out what was "bad." I was optimistic that my positive energy would rub off and that I could rescue her from her gloom. I was so hurt that we could not save our relationship. The truth is that I have had many challenges in my life, and although she thought "only good things happened" to me, it was not true. The success I have is the success I have earned. I know that my "attitude of gratitude" has had a significant impact on my outlook, as well as my ability to let things go that interfered with my path to success.

I had to learn to "let go" of what I thought our friendship was. It was obviously different for her than it was for me. I still hurt from that loss. Letting go has been one of the hardest struggles of my life. I've learned that there are people who come into your life at different seasons; you need them at certain points in your life, but then sometimes that friendship has served its purpose and you are meant to move on.

I think sometimes people get into a situation where they hold on to things from the past that keep them from going forward. It could be a friendship, or it could be a material possession, and either way it might not be healthy. It was hard for me to say goodbye to people, and also to possessions. It was especially hard to let go of things connected to people I was close to—something that would remind me of a friend was meaningful and sentimental. But being too sentimental can keep you from fully enjoying the present, from fully appreciating the people who are present in your life here and now. Holding on to a past friendship or relationship, or a material possession that reminds us of someone we loved and have lost, can also keep us from completing tasks or achieving goals, because it takes our focus from the present.

Fears or preconceived notions can also be very challenging to let go of. A friend recently shared with me an experience that helped her let go of a preconceived notion. Before becoming a mother, she feared having a handicapped child and thought it would be the end of the world and would mean a life full of hardship and heartache. She was very relieved when her daughter was born without any handicaps or disabilities. Many years later, while on vacation with her daughter, she had opportunity to sit on a ride in a theme park directly across from a mother with a handicapped daughter. This woman's daughter was physically an adult, but clearly had the mental capacity of a child. Initially my friend felt a bit uncomfortable, but as she observed the interaction between the mother and the daughter, she was moved by the great love that they clearly shared. She was surprised by the mother's joy and delight as she enjoyed the theme park with her daughter. Her joy was infectious and almost tangible. The bond between mother and daughter was a beautiful thing to experience. It was clear that the mother viewed her child as a blessing and not as a burden. This experience completely changed my friend's concept of what love looked like. It was liberating.

As I work on this book, I am reminded of "letting go of perfection." I have been trying to write this book for a couple of years. I had lots of ideas for it, and it's gone through many different evolutions in my mind. But it seemed as if I could never write it, because it just wasn't perfect. I had to let go of my fear of being judged for revealing vulnerabilities. I had to keep in mind *why* I wanted to write the book in the first place. I want the book to be a practical tool to help people stay happy as they age. I feel so privileged that people trust me to help them, and I am eager to educate people about healthy alternatives to help slow down the aging process. When I focused on this goal, I was able to actually write something that I truly believe is going to be meaningful and make a difference. But I had to let go of the preconceived notion that my first book was going to be perfect.

I also had to let go of the idea that I could do it by myself and get help from a team with the skills and experience and time to help me make it happen. I had to let them figure out the details—*What will the cover look like? Who is going to edit it? How am I going to market it?* We all need help, and when we recognize that we need help, we're able to accomplish our goals and make something that we can be proud of.

I remember reading a study while I was a second-year medical student at UC Davis that described successful people. I was surprised to read that the most successful people recognized they needed help, and then asked for help when they needed it. I think that one important aspect of letting go is understanding what you are strong in and where your weaknesses lie. Sometimes we have limitations that keep us from achieving our goal, and if we don't recognize what they are, then we don't realize what we need to let go of, or we don't get the help that we need in order to succeed.

A closing thought: I've learned that sometimes you have to let go of being in control in order to genuinely have control of a situation.

ACTION:

REFLECT ON LETTING GO

What are you holding on to that, if you would let go of, your life would improve? It could be material possessions, expectations, perceptions, ideas, emotions, or relationships. Reflect and journal. Decide on at least one thing to let go of. Then mark your calendar to reflect again a month from now, and see how letting go has helped you.

NOTES:

1. Hewitt, Paul L., and Dennis G. Dyck. "Perfectionism, stress, and vulnerability to depression." *Cognitive Therapy and Research* 10, no. 1 (1986): 137–142. **http://link.springer.com/article/10.1007/BF01173389**

2. Burmark, Lynell, and Lou Fournier. *Enlighten Up! An Educator's Guide to Stress-Free Living.* Association for Supervision and Curriculum Development, 1703 North Beauregard Street, Alexandria, VA 22311-1714 (ASCD product no. 102106), 2003. **http://eric.ed.gov/?id=ED476075**

3. Timpano, Kiara R., Meghan E. Keough, Lara Traeger, and Norman B. Schmidt. "General life stress and hoarding: Examining the role of emotional tolerance." *International Journal of Cognitive Therapy* 4, no. 3 (2011): 263–279. **http://guilfordjournals.com/doi/abs/10.1521/ijct.2011.4.3.263**

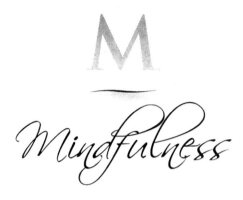

Mindfulness

"*Do not dwell in the past. Do not dream of the future. Concentrate the mind on the present moment.*"

—Gautama Buddha

Mindfulness is about being in the present moment. It's having an increased awareness and understanding of your thoughts, your feelings, and your environment. At the same time, there is no label, attachment, or judgment.

The busyness of our everyday lives tends to keep our minds in the future. *What's happening next?* And mindfulness brings us into the present.

As busy women with both families and careers, we're always struggling to find the balance in our professional and personal lives. Sometimes our to-do list distracts us from doing what we need to do here and now, because we're worried about checking off the things on our lists, making sure that we get through our day. We're always thinking and planning ahead to keep up, and that distracts us from enjoying the present.

I'm challenged by being a multitasker. I've been known to have three computers or screens open at one time—paying bills on one, checking email on another, and writing on a third. During one such multitasking session, my second son was trying to get my attention. I was engrossed in my work and didn't look up from the computer screens, and my son said emphatically, "Mama, I want you to listen with your *eyes*." It made me stop what I was doing, and once again I learned something profound from one of my children.

He wanted to connect with me. At that moment I realized the importance of being present; that when someone who is important to you wants to communicate and connect with you, giving your attention and being present is key and should not be neglected. I thought of other times when I hadn't looked up from my computer and answered his questions or addressed his needs—all those times when I didn't fully connect, and missed out on those opportunities. When you "listen with your eyes," it's very powerful. And you can't listen with your eyes if you're texting, or looking at your phone or your computer screen. Try listening more with your eyes and making that full connection.

For me, having a regular meditation practice helps clear the clutter in my brain. It helps keep me from being distracted. It kind of "reboots" my brain—like a computer needs to be rebooted, because when you have too many things open and running, it starts getting sluggish. That's how my brain feels sometimes when I'm trying to think about too many things. Meditation helps me to take a break from my to-do list, from all the tasks at hand and my responsibilities. It helps increase mental clarity and create inner peace. And when you have that inner peace, you're going to be more productive.

There's a study from a Harvard researcher that shows how mindfulness can help to combat stress.[1] In the study, the researcher describes many positive aspects of mindfulness. It can enhance body awareness, increase your sense of self, and regulate emotion. The evidence in this study suggests that mindfulness actually creates physiological changes in the brain. The most outstanding takeaway from this study was how mindful meditation helped people cope with stressful situations in everyday life. It helped people to feel more centered, to gain insight into their purpose for living, and for doing what they needed to do. Most importantly, mindfulness helped them focus on the present moment and removed the distractions that were keeping them from completing a goal or task.

When we introduce mindfulness into our life, let's try to think about how we can do it on a daily basis. For example, whenever we are feeling stressed or anxious, we can be mindful and aware of that moment, of that anxiety; and instead of passing judgment, just acknowledge it and then let go of it. At the end of this chapter, I will describe how to do a simple meditation, how to use belly breathing to help reduce anxiety, and how to practice Loving-Kindness Meditation. The ideal is to be consistent with meditation. Start with five minutes, once a day. The more you meditate, the better you become at meditating. You start to recognize physiological changes in your body, such as lower blood pressure and better sleep.

My husband had ongoing problems falling asleep, and instead of reaching for prescription drugs, we meditated together. It was challenging in the beginning, but with practice he was able to fall asleep like a baby. Some days he had to also take melatonin—which is a natural hormone our brain makes when we sleep—but his sleep has improved significantly with meditation practice.

You can also practice mindfulness on a daily basis by simply being more aware of your surroundings and people you love. Try looking at your world through the eyes of a five-year-old child, where everything is seen with awe. You could even do one of the spontaneous things that kids do—like chasing butterflies, dancing in the rain, and running through the puddles.

Remember a time in your life when you didn't judge, when everything you saw amazed you, and you just appreciated the beauty. Remember when you marveled at a new idea, or looked forward to an upcoming event or interaction, and there was no judgment or label on it. You just accepted the feeling, the idea, as it was, and enjoyed the experience of the moment.

You might also decide that you want to do a full-day meditation or a weekend meditation. For those who want intense practice, there are 3-day to 7-day meditation retreats, which take more investment of time and money, but can be life-changing for some. However you choose to do it, practice meditation and mindfulness in some way. And remember, to be mindful is to be aware, and to accept without judgment.

Meditation basics for beginners: five-minute power meditation

Find a quiet place where you can be still and free from distractions. For example, if you're at work, go to your car or into an empty office. Make sure the door is locked, put a "do not disturb" sign out, or somehow let people know not to interrupt you. If you're at home, find a quiet room, or maybe a spot outside. The place you choose should be at a comfortable temperature for you. You're going to want to turn your cellphone off so you won't be interrupted by calls.

You can set a timer if you like, if it helps you relax and be less concerned or anxious about the time, which can be distracting to some people.

Sit comfortably, either with your legs crossed or in a chair with your legs uncrossed. Your hands can be on your lap, or just hanging down at your sides, but should be in a relaxed position. Make sure that your body overall is fully relaxed. Sometimes I meditate in my bed before going to sleep, and I lie flat on my back, with my hands outstretched parallel to my body. The goal is to find a comfortable position where you can be still.

As you start the meditation, close your eyes and become aware of anything that's uncomfortable in your body, any kind of pain. Try to dissipate that discomfort by noticing it, acknowledging it, and then letting it be. Take a deep breath in, and then as you breathe out, imagine the pain leaving your body. The goal is to replace your thoughts with focus on your breaths.

When you practice meditation, you are practicing mindfulness without judgment. You're entering a place where you're not judging any thoughts or feelings. You're just being present. The goal is to achieve stillness.

Breathe in deeply, and breathe out slowly. You can start by taking a deep breath in through your nostrils, and then breathing out through your mouth. You are very mindful of each breath. Breathe in as you count to three, and then breathe out slowly, for at least a count of three. Acknowledge the breaths coming in and going out. Try not to think about anything other than your breath. If a thought comes into your head, imagine that you are breathing out that thought.

Belly Breathing Technique

Belly breathing is a good tool to use if you feel anxious, or if you have a repetitive thought that you cannot get rid of or be at peace with. Inhale deeply and slowly for a count of three while trying to push your belly out. You can put your hand on your belly and as you breathe in, make sure you're pushing your belly out. And as you breathe out, feel your belly contract and pull back in. It may take some practice, so don't be frustrated or judge yourself on how you do it. You get the same benefit with breathing deeply, whether or not you do belly breathing. The goal is to practice deep breathing and focus on your breath.

Loving-Kindness Meditation (A Buddhist Tradition)

In this meditation, you start with nurturing love for yourself and then move to wishing love and wellness to all beings. In Loving-Kindness Meditation, your thoughts are intentional and you acknowledge that each person is precious.

Start with a comfortable, unrestricted position. Relax and close your eyes.

First stage: Embrace loving-kindness toward yourself. You can imagine rays of light or something that gives you peace of mind. Recite a positive affirmation to yourself: "May I be compassionate." "May I be wise." "May I be happy."

Second stage: Shift your focus from self-love into sending loving-kindness to someone you love. Visualize that person and recite: "May they feel love." "May they feel peace."

Third stage: After a few minutes, focus your attention toward a "neutral person" such as a clerk at a store or a stranger that has passed by. Visualize that person and recite: "May they be wise." "May they be strong."

Fourth stage: Shift your attention to someone who you find difficult or unfriendly. If this is challenging, try to think of that person in a vulnerable position, such as in pain or in need of your help. Or you can focus on someone who you know is suffering. Visualize them and recite: "May they have wellness." "May they be happy."

Last stage: Finally, send loving kindness to all beings: "May they have peace." "May they have joy." "May they have love."

ACTION:

PRACTICE ONE OF THE MEDITATION
TECHNIQUES DESCRIBED

Download and listen to one of the mp3 meditation recordings I have provided on my website: www.drmelindasilva.com.

Choose a meditation technique to practice at least five minutes daily.

NOTES:

1. Hölzel, Britta K., Sara W. Lazar, Tim Gard, Zev Schuman-Olivier, David R. Vago, and Ulrich Ott. "How does mindfulness meditation work? Proposing mechanisms of action from a conceptual and neural perspective." *Perspectives on Psychological Science* 6, no. 6 (2011): 537–559. http://pps.sagepub.com/content/6/6/537.short

N

New

"*Learn to love. Love to learn.*
So that you may live the life that you yearn."

—Rico Dasheem

There is research that shows that if you keep your brain engaged by learning new things or doing new activities, experiencing new thoughts and new ideas, you actually enhance the neural plasticity of your brain. This means you can maintain or create new neural connections, which has the result of slowing down the aging process of your brain! Cognitive training, or "exercising your brain" if you will, may actually enhance neural and cognitive function as we age.[1]

Challenge your brain to something new in whatever way works for you. It can be as simple as taking a different route when you're driving home, or trying a new recipe. Or you could take up a new hobby, or take a class or series of classes. Engaging your mind in activities outside of what you routinely do increases the cognitive function in your brain.

I think of myself as a student of learning, a student of life. I went into the field of medicine because I knew that within it I would always have the opportunity to learn something new, because the field is ever-changing. Having the attitude of being a student of life keeps your mind open to experiences that enrich your life. As we age, it is healthy for us to either try something new or reacquaint ourselves with things that are familiar to us but that we haven't done for a while. For example, I used to play the piano. I loved playing the piano, and I keep saying that I want to play the piano again. So that would be an example of something that I could reintroduce into my life that would be new in a way, and yet I wouldn't have to start from scratch.

I also want to be more creative and take sculpting or painting classes. Just recently I went with some friends to a "paint and wine" event, where in a couple of hours we were actually able to paint something to take home that we could be proud of—and we had fun in the process. Doing simple things like that doesn't take a lot of time or money, but gives you a chance to express yourself creatively—which exercises a part of your brain that you might not use on a regular basis.

I'm reminded of an encounter I had with one of my mentors. He was one of the first doctors I worked with when I started at Kaiser in 1998 and he was intelligent, smart, and a very competent and compassionate physician. He has since retired, and not long ago I saw him in front of a restaurant. We hadn't seen each other for a few years, and I was very excited to see him, but I could tell from the look on his face that he didn't even recognize me. It was as if he looked straight through me, his eyes without expression. His lovely wife was sitting next to him, and you could see the sadness on her face. She didn't have to tell me that he was affected with dementia. His blank stare made it evident.

That emptiness that I saw in his eyes was shocking and frightening. It reminded me of the reality of dementia, and how it can hit us unexpectedly. It reinforced my determination to guard my brain from cognitive decline. I've seen firsthand how dementia has devastated families. The worst thing about dementia is that you are not aware of the changes going on in your brain. Your family suffers so much, and they just become a distant memory. Who do we become if we have no memory of who we are or who we love?

There's important research from the *Journal of American Medical Association* (JAMA), which shows that the beta amyloid plaques that accumulate between the nerve cells create an increased risk of Alzheimer's.[2] The JAMA article showed that patients who had plenty of early or midlife cognitive activity—meaning they stimulated their brain with reading, writing, learning, etc.—had a lower tendency toward the beta amyloid plaques building up. This decreased their risk of Alzheimer's. Another article that came out in the *New England Journal of Medicine* showed that when participants did leisure activities, this was also associated with a lower risk of dementia.[3] Reading, playing chess, bridge, or board games, playing musical instruments, and dancing, all were associated with reduced risk of dementia.

Other activities that stimulate the brain are doing crossword or other puzzles, or playing games such as those found on www.Lumosity.com.[4] Also, being bilingual appears to delay the onset of Alzheimer's. Staying mentally active and productive has a positive effect on longevity. A French study showed that retiring at an older age decreases the incidence of dementia.[5]

There are also studies that show that the risk of developing Alzheimer's disease is greater when people have cardiovascular problems such as diabetes, high blood pressure, high cholesterol, or stroke.[6] Obesity appears to raise the risks of dementia, and diabetes increases the risk of dementia considerably. Alzheimer's has been called "Diabetes Type 3" because the insulin resistance and/or insulin deficiency can happen selectively in the brain, leading to cognitive impairment and memory issues.

The diet that appears to protect the brain from Alzheimer's or dementia is the Mediterranean diet, which is also heart-healthy.

The main source of fat in the Mediterranean diet is olive oil. The hallmark of the diet is to eat plenty of fruits and vegetables, legumes, and high amounts of fresh fish or seafood. It is also important to minimize red meat and dairy. Moderate consumption of red wine also seems to be protective for a vascular type of dementia.

Supplements that improve mental ability and decrease the risk of dementia are omega-3 fatty acids,[7] lipoic acid,[8] and vitamin D.[9] Eating fish at least once a week also reduces mild cognitive impairment, which is the first step toward reducing dementia.

Research from the Alzheimer's Association shows, based on results from autopsies, that 80 percent of people who had Alzheimer's also had cardiovascular disease. So keeping your heart healthy is also important to keeping your brain healthy.

To reduce your risk of dementia: Don't smoke, or at least decrease smoking. Exercise regularly. Keep your body at a healthy weight. Keep blood sugar under control by focusing on a whole food diet. Eat more fruits and vegetables. Exercise your mind. And make sure you get plenty of good sleep.[10]

A strong heart and strong mind work together in helping you age gracefully.

ACTION:

TRY SOMETHING NEW!

What is something new you can sign up for that will exercise your brain? Is there a class you can take to learn something new that you're interested in? A new activity or craft you can try? Write down a few ideas now, and sign up within the next few days or week.

NOTES:

1. Park, Denise C., and Gérard N. Bischof. "The aging mind: neuroplasticity in response to cognitive training." *Dialogues in Clinical Neuroscience* 15, no. 1 (2013): 109.
http://www.ncbi.nlm.nih.gov/pubmed/23576894

2. Landau, Susan M., Shawn M. Marks, Elizabeth C. Mormino, Gil D. Rabinovici, Hwamee Oh, James P. O'Neil, Robert S. Wilson, and William J. Jagust. "Association of lifetime cognitive engagement and low ß-amyloid deposition." *Archives of Neurology* 69, no. 5 (2012): 623–629. http://archneur.jamanetwork.com/article.aspx?articleid=1149704

3. Verghese, Joe, Richard B. Lipton, Mindy J. Katz, Charles B. Hall, Carol A. Derby, Gail Kuslansky, Anne F. Ambrose, Martin Sliwinski, and Herman Buschke. "Leisure activities and the risk of dementia in the elderly." *New England Journal of Medicine* 348, no. 25 (2003): 2508–2516. http://www.nejm.org/doi/full/10.1056/NEJMoa022252

4. Hardy, Joseph, David Drescher, Kunal Sarkar, Gregory Kellett, and Michael Scanlon. "Enhancing visual attention and working memory with a web-based cognitive training program." *A Lumos Labs White Paper* (2011). http://static.sl.lumosity.com/pdf/hardy_drescher_sarkar_kellet_scanlon_2011.pdf

5. Dufouil, Carole, Edwige Pereira, Geneviève Chêne, M. Maria Glymour, Annick Alpérovitch, Elodie Saubusse, Mathilde Risse-Fleury et al. "Older age at retirement is associated with decreased risk of dementia." *European Journal of Epidemiology* (2014): 353–61. http://www.ncbi.nlm.nih.gov/pubmed/24791704

6. Suzanne, M., and Jack R. Wands. "Alzheimer's disease is type 3 diabetes—evidence reviewed." *Journal of Diabetes Science and Technology* 2, no. 6 (2008): 1101-1113. http://www.ncbi.nlm.nih.gov/pmc/articles/PMC2769828/

7. Hjorth E, Zhu M, Toro VC, Vedin I, Palmblad J, Cederholm T, Freund-Levi Y, Faxen-Irving G, Wahlund LO, Basun H, Eriksdotter M, Schultzberg M. "Omega-3 fatty acids enhance phagocytosis of Alzheimer's disease-related amyloid-β42 by human microglia and decrease inflammatory markers." *Journal of Alzheimer's Disease* 35, no. 4 (2013): 697–713. http://www.ncbi.nlm.nih.gov/pubmed/23481688

8. Maczurek, Annette, Klaus Hager, Marlene Kenklies, Matt Sharman, Ralph Martins, Jürgen Engel, David A. Carlson, and Gerald Münch. "Lipoic acid as an anti-inflammatory and neuroprotective treatment for Alzheimer's disease." *Advanced Drug Delivery Reviews* 60, no. 13 (2008): 1463–1470 http://www.sciencedirect.com/science/article/pii/S0169409X08001592

9. Annweiler, Cédric, and Olivier Beauchet. "Possibility of a new anti-Alzheimer's disease pharmaceutical composition combining memantine and vitamin D." *Drugs and Aging* 29, no. 2 (2012): 81–91. http://link.springer.com/article/10.2165/11597550-000000000-00000#page-1

10. Prevention of Alzheimer's disease and dementia: http://www.medicalnewstoday.com/articles/263769.php

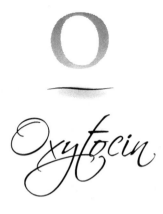

O

Oxytocin

"Good sex is like good bridge. If you don't have a good partner, you'd better have a good hand."

—Mae West

Oxytocin, what I call "the big O," is mainly known for its role in reproductive medicine. Oxytocin is released in large amounts during labor as well as breastfeeding. It is produced in the hypothalamus and secreted by the pituitary glands. This hormone is responsible for the letdown reflex during breastfeeding, and it is postulated that it is not only important for the production of milk, but also the bonding between mother and baby.

Oxytocin is known as "the bonding hormone." It is also released in large amounts during social bonding and orgasm (the other big "O").

There are many beneficial effects of oxytocin.[1,2,3] It helps to relax muscles and to decrease blood pressure. It has been shown to elevate mood and decrease anxiety. It's also required for proper muscle tissue regeneration, and prevents skeletal muscle aging. It can enhance sexual pleasure and it has been postulated to trigger multiple orgasms, particularly in women.

There is exciting research that shows that oxytocin can increase longevity by having a cardioprotective effect on the heart. A ten-year study in the south of Wales examined the relationship between orgasm and mortality, and the results showed that mortality risk was 50 percent lower in the group with high orgasmic frequency, compared to the group with low orgasmic frequency. So sexual activity seems to have a protective effect on men's health. The statistic they gave was at least 100 orgasms per year. More sex has a correlation with increased longevity. So, the bottom line is that sex is good for you![4]

People with higher oxytocin levels tend to be happier and more sociable. Oxytocin decreases inhibition, and people with enough of it have better interactions with others, including increased trust and decreased anxiety. On the other hand, people with lower oxytocin levels generally would rather be alone and avoid human contact.

Oxytocin is triggered by human touch, such as kissing or hugging. Also, when someone even looks at a picture of somebody that they're attracted to, especially someone they love, oxytocin levels will increase naturally.

There are many ways someone can increase their oxytocin levels naturally. Romantic love, or even a mother's love, can boost it. A hug, a massage, positive social interactions, being at a party, or going on a date, can all help. Looking at pictures of loved ones, listening to music, singing, and physical exercise are also ways to increase oxytocin levels. And the most popular way is to have an orgasm.

One of the happiest patients I treated was Nancy M., who recently had an orgasm for the first time in her life at 40 years old! She initially came to see me because she was tired and was struggling with weight gain. When I questioned her about libido, she was very timid and uncomfortable talking about sex. After I balanced her hormones, she started to feel better, and her libido and interest in sex increased. However, she was still frustrated because she could not have an orgasm. We gave her oxytocin, and soon after that she not only had the first orgasm in her life, but multiple orgasms.

While oxytocin might be touted as a party drug, it is important to know that it is a prescription drug which is available from a pharmacy, requiring a doctor's prescription. It can be given as a tablet or as a pill sublingual, and newer methods include intranasal application.

It is very common for me to hear my female patients, especially after age 35, confess to decreased libido. I ask all my patients about sex, because in my clinical practice, I have noticed that my happiest patients are those who have intimacy and satisfying sex with their partner. It is not a coincidence that many relationship challenges occur when people are in their 40s and 50s, experiencing the so-called "midlife crisis." People can start having breakdowns in communication when there are emotional and physical changes in their bodies, like fatigue and vaginal dryness due to hormonal decline. People get impatient with each other when they don't feel well, and wrongly blame each other. I work with a lot of couples and help them to increase their sex drive and rediscover their intimacy. It is very satisfying for me when couples tell me that I have saved their marriage.

I was appalled when Nancy M. told me about her visit to her previous doctor. When Nancy finally had enough courage to share her issues with decreased interest in sex and lack of orgasm, her OB-GYN told her that she must not love her husband enough. Her OB-GYN told her she should just lie there and have sex with her husband because that was her duty as a wife. This made Nancy feel so guilty, and she blamed herself for not wanting to have sex with her husband. She was starting to believe that it was her fault, or that there was something wrong with her, because she didn't want to have sex.

Fortunately, she shared this experience with her friend, who encouraged her to come see me and get her hormones evaluated. The reality is, decrease in libido is a normal process that can happen to women when their hormones are out of balance. As we age, our hormones decline, and with the declining hormones, certain functions in our body don't work optimally. Without proper hormonal balance your vaginal walls can be drier and thinner. Sexual relations can cause friction burn, and even small tears and bleeding, when there is not enough lubrication. Painful sex is not fun and can definitely decrease libido. Even without physical changes, decreased hormones can cause decline in sexual desire. And if oxytocin levels are decreased, intensity or frequency of orgasm may be diminished. It is important to remember that hormone decline has nothing to do with how *much* you love someone, but it can affect *how* you love them.

There are other supplements and "tools" that can be used to help women reach orgasm, with or without a partner. Special topical creams to increase libido and orgasm, such as "scream cream," can be rubbed directly on the clitoris and vaginal opening. These are prescription creams dispensed from a compounding pharmacy. The FDA has approved a sexual device to improve sexual dysfunction in women called EROS clitoral therapy device.[5] It is for women with female sexual arousal disorder and helps them achieve climax by increasing blood flow and direct stimulation to the clitoris. This device requires a prescription.

From my clinical experience, there are other devices that work to increase orgasm for women which are much less expensive and do not require a prescription. A great tool is a "personal massager," available from University Compounding Pharmacy. It can be used all over the body. One of my patients claimed it "changed her life" and increased her desire to be with her husband when it was used in their sexual encounters. For further info, please discuss with Dr. Silva during your hormone consultation. It's important for our health and happiness as we age to have satisfying sex lives. Oxytocin can be an integral component, and there are many ways to enhance it naturally, as noted above. For those who don't have a sexual partner, keep in mind that self-stimulation and self-pleasure can help increase oxytocin—it doesn't have to be someone else's touch. Self-massage, or touching your own body in a nonsexual way, can also help.

Even reading a steamy novel helps. Women all over the nation who put *Fifty Shades of Grey* on the bestselling list were increasing their oxytocin levels naturally.

ACTION:

GET TO KNOW YOUR O

Do one or more of the following within the next week or two:

* Read a romantic or steamy novel.

* Get a deep muscle massage, or a sensual massage with body oils.

* Visit your local adult store and buy a sex toy.

* Spend some time getting acquainted with your personal erogenous zones, and which areas of your body and private parts give you the most pleasure. When you know what gives you pleasure, you are then better able to communicate this to your partner. Don't be shy—share your desires with your partner. It will increase your intimacy and result in more satisfying sexual encounters.

NOTES:

1. Elabd, Christian, Wendy Cousin, Pavan Upadhyayula, Robert Y. Chen, Marc S. Chooljian, Ju Li, Sunny Kung, Kevin P. Jiang, and Irina M. Conboy. "Oxytocin is an age-specific circulating hormone that is necessary for muscle maintenance and regeneration." *Nature Communications* 5 (2014). **http://www.nature.com/ncomms/2014/140610/ncomms5082/full/ ncomms5082.html**

2. Magon, Navneet, and Sanjay Kalra. "The orgasmic history of oxytocin: Love, lust, and labor." *Indian Journal of Endocrinology and Metabolism* 15, no. Suppl3 (2011): S156.
http://www.ncbi.nlm.nih.gov/pubmed/22029018

3. Carmichael, Marie S., Richard Humbert, Jean Dixen, Glenn Palmisano, Walter Greenleaf, and Julian M. Davidson. "Plasma Oxytocin Increases in the Human Sexual Response." *The Journal of Clinical Endocrinology & Metabolism* 64, no. 1 (1987): 27–31.
http://www.ncbi.nlm.nih.gov/pubmed/3782434

4. Smith, George Davey, Stephen Frankel, and John Yarnell. "Sex and death: are they related? Findings from the Caerphilly cohort study." *BMJ* 315, no. 7123 (1997): 1641–1644.
http://www.bmj.com/content/315/7123/1641?goto=reply

5. Josefson, Debbie. "FDA approves device for female sexual dysfunction." *British Medical Journal* 320, no. 7247 (2000): 1427.
http://www.ncbi.nlm.nih.gov/pmc/articles/PMC1127636/

P

Priorities and Productivity

"*If I had to embrace a definition of success, it would be that success is making the best choices we can ... and accepting them.*"

—Sheryl Sandberg, COO of Facebook and Author of *Lean In*

I believe that the key to productivity is prioritizing what's important to you in life, understanding your limitations, and focusing your energies on your priorities. One motto I live by is: Do what you do best, and outsource the rest.

Balancing my professional and personal life has always been a challenge. I married my best friend during medical school. Medicine can be a very time-consuming and stressful practice. Multiply that stress by two and it can be overwhelming for some couples to focus on a relationship. Fortunately our marriage worked, because my husband and I had a relationship that started with a strong friendship that matured into an enduring love. The fact that we shared the same values about work and family was crucial.

I became pregnant with my first child during my fourth year of medical school. I chose to defer my internship (first year after medical school), because I knew that being a mother was going to be *the* most important job of my life. It was my priority. I have never regretted staying home during my son's first year of life. My colleagues who were career-centered gasped at the idea of taking a year off. It was a fork in the road for me; the first of many things I learned about what it would take to balance motherhood and marriage with my career.

Many doctors would agree that completing their internship is one of the most stressful and challenging years of their medical career. This is a pivotal year, where you become responsible for the health and well-being of those who seek your advice and care. The year our first son was born, my husband was an intern. When my husband was at home during his internship year, he was exhausted and trying to catch up on much-needed sleep. It was difficult for me, since I felt like a single mom at times. Then when my son was a year old, my husband had to take a bigger role in raising him while I was doing *my* internship. That was very stressful for my husband. Sometimes when I was spending a night on call at the hospital, my husband would bring our son to me before his bedtime so that I could kiss him goodnight, sing to him, and ideally he would fall asleep. My husband would take him home asleep, but he would often wake up in the middle of the night and cry for me, and that was very hard for my husband. I feel blessed that my mom was able to step in and help us during this time. It was nice to have that help from someone we could trust and rely on.

The hospital had a daycare facility right off the parking lot, and I still remember the first day I left my son there. He was two and a half years old at the time, vibrant, expressive, and happy. As I walked out of the daycare, I tried not to look back. I saw him following me and he walked up to the fence, peering through the railing, reached toward me and said, "I love you, Mama." I remember the guilt that pierced my heart, but I also knew he was secure and happy and I felt confident he knew I was coming back for him. I hid behind one of the cars in the parking lot and took a last peek at him. He was still standing there, his face against the railing, now holding the fence with his chubby hands, his big brown eyes searching the parking lot. My tears fell onto my white lab coat and I knew this would be my life.

After our early years of marriage, I had confidence that our relationship was going to survive. For a marriage to endure the stress of internship is a great sign, but to survive two years of internship is a sign your relationship will endure to the end. Fortunately, the 100+ hour work week is not as commonplace now as it was back then, over 20 years ago. Recognizing the brutality of that work schedule, hospitals have changed regulations to limit the number of hours worked for patient safety and physician sanity.

Now I have four children, and my own medical practice, and balancing my life and priorities has become even more challenging. My priority, as I determined those many years ago, remains being a mother.

I have the privilege of doing a weekly parenting segment on our local television station, Fox 5, called "Ask the Moms." On one of the segments we discussed the controversy over an interview that Indra K. Nooyi, the CEO of Pepsi, gave *The Atlantic*, where she said that women can't have it all. She felt that if you asked her daughters what kind of mother she was, they would likely say she was not a good mother. She felt guilty about not participating in a lot of school activities, about not being the ideal mother she would have liked to be. It is very typical for women to have that kind of guilt when they have a career and they're trying to juggle professional and personal lives. While I appreciated her candor and sympathized with her guilt about not being a good mother, I happen to think that women *can* have it all—but, you can't have it all, *all the time*.

I wear a lot of hats. I'm a mother, wife, daughter, sister, aunt, niece, friend, and doctor. I play the different roles in my life at different times during the day, week, or month. On any given day, I will set my priorities for that day, and I accept that some days I will be a better doctor than a mother. Sometimes I will be a better mother than a doctor. We have to make the best choices we can to fulfill our priorities, our goals, and our obligations.

I can't make it to all of my kids' school events, and yes, I used to feel guilty about that. I make it to the significant events, and will ask my kids which events are a "must go" and rearrange my work schedule to fit those in. When my kids are recognized for their achievements, I am the proud parent in the front row, camera in hand! If my children are disappointed that I can't make a particular event at school, I will set aside some time on the weekend shortly after that event to spend time with them. I actually put it on my calendar, just as I would any other appointment. My kids *know* that they are a priority to me, and I'm proud to say that, and that's what I want to focus on. They also know I have great responsibility at my work, and that on some days that will take priority. But they know my work is never more important than my role as their mother.

In order to attend to my priorities, even to keep up with different ones on different days, I have to get help and support from others. This is where I focus on what I do best and don't feel guilty about delegating or outsourcing the rest. I can't do everything. My priorities include feeding my family and having a clean house and clean clothes; so I pay somebody to do the laundry and clean my house. When I come home from work I'm not going to spend time doing those chores, because I want to spend quality time with my family. Some people will pay somebody to do grocery shopping for them, or they do it online and get it delivered. I happen to particularly like grocery shopping, because I love choosing food! It's a priority for me to have my family eat home-cooked meals, but it's not a priority for me to cook *all* of those meals for them. I will buy what we need to prepare the food and make the menu of what I want to be cooked and served, but I won't necessarily spend the time cooking. I enjoy cooking, but sometimes it does not make my list of priorities that day. My daughter likes to cook with me on the weekend, so we make it a family event and a way that I can spend time with her.

We are only truly productive when we are focusing on our priorities. Managing our time well both helps us get done what we need to do and helps to reduce stress. Reducing stress increases longevity. It gets harder, as we get older, to multitask—so it becomes all the more important to manage our time and focus on our priorities.

Prioritizing and managing our time—really, managing our *lives*—is especially relevant for people in what we call the "sandwich generation," people in their 30s or 40s who are responsible both for bringing up their own children and for taking care of their aging parents. This is a time when there may be more competing priorities and potential for more stress if you don't have available resources in place to help you. There's a study that shows that women are more likely than men to have caregiver strain—stress from taking care of their parents at the same time as taking care of their kids and their own lives. That's because women tend to devote more hours per week, compared to men, to the specific activities related to taking care of their children and their parents, as well as chores around the house.[1]

Productivity has been linked with longevity in some studies. In the village of Ogimi in Japan, almost every elderly woman in the village is productive, active in the business of weaving—which is an important part of their culture. These elderly women play a key role in the production process, and they receive respect and honor from their community, as well as wages for their labor. The study showed that having an active engagement with life and work helped these women to be healthy and productive members of society.[2]

Being productive is important, and has implications as to how we age. We need to be productive in order to age strong. At the same time, too much "productivity" can cause stress, and we need to keep stress in check. We have to find the balance, and clarifying our priorities helps us do that.

Remember when you're clarifying your priorities that it's personal, and there are no "right" or "wrong" priorities. My family is my priority, and many mothers may say the same. For others, priorities might include careers, pets, or friendships. For some it might be a hobby like painting or dancing. The key is that *you* know what *your* priority is. And that you accept it, and then create your schedule and life based around what's important to you.

ACTION:

PRIORITIZE

List your top three priorities in life.

Then take a look at both your checkbook/bank account and your calendar, and see what these say about your priorities. What are the three things you *actually* spend a majority of your time and money on? Do these match your desired priorities?

If not, decide on what changes you are going to make. Schedule time in your calendar for your true priorities.

NOTES:

1. Duxbury, Linda, Christopher Higgins, and Rob Smart. "Elder care and the impact of caregiver strain on the health of employed caregivers." *Work: A Journal of Prevention, Assessment and Rehabilitation* 40, no. 1 (2011): 29–40. **http://iospress.metapress.com/content/b20u211561713507/**

2. Willcox, D. Craig, Bradley J. Willcox, Jay Sokolovsky, and Seizo Sakihara. "The cultural context of 'successful aging' among older women weavers in a northern Okinawan village: The role of productive activity." *Journal of Cross-Cultural Gerontology* 22, no. 2 (2007): 137–165. **http://link.springer.com/article/10.1007/s10823-006-9032-0**

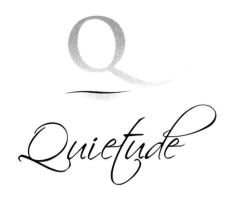

Quietude

"*A good laugh and a long sleep are the two best cures in a doctor's book.*"

—Irish Proverb

qui·e·tude

ˈkwīəˌt(y)o͞od/

noun

a state of stillness, calmness, and quiet in a person or place.

Quietude is a state of being which helps us to get good quality sleep. It is absolute stillness of mind and body. People who have difficulty sleeping need to aim for quietude prior to falling into slumber.

Sleep has significant implications for our health, effects which are often underrated. Sleep is very important for health of body as well as mind—it's the time when both can rejuvenate.

In the book *The Promise of Sleep,* there is extensive research showing that healthful sleep is a more important factor in predicting longevity than diet, exercise, or heredity.[1] Everybody talks about the healthful habits of the right diet and exercise, but you rarely hear people talk about making sure to get a good night's rest. Sometimes it is taken for granted. Many people will sacrifice sleep in order to finish their to-do list. I used to be one of those people who would burn the midnight oil, answering email or catching up on my reading long after my family had gone to bed. When I completed my fellowship in Functional and Regenerative Medicine, I learned the importance of sleep in rejuvenating the mind and body. It is very apparent to me now that poor sleep ruins an otherwise good day.

Notable research on sleep by the American Cancer Society in 1982 studied the sleeping habits of more than 1,000,000 men and women from 30 to 102 years of age. One of the results of the study was that people who consistently slept either less than 4.5 hours or more than 8.5 hours had significant increased mortality risk. The best survival rates were found among the participants who slept seven hours on average per night. The study also found that prescription sleeping pill use was associated with increased mortality. In conclusion: better sleep, the right amount of sleep, and sleep without chemical aids were factors in longer life expectancy.[2]

The average adult should optimally get seven hours of sleep. For teenagers and adults over 65, having closer to nine hours of sleep is ideal.

Insomnia and sleep disturbances are a common reason for patients to seek my help. Recently, I reviewed a note regarding my patient Marcela, who was evaluated in the ER. Marcela showed up at the ER because she had not been able to sleep for three days. The initial complaint was insomnia. Marcela proceeded to tell the doctor in the ER that "Jesus was speaking to her through her television" and spoke of other psychotic delusions. After psychiatric evaluation, she was found to be bipolar. Fortunately, instead of being prescribed a sleeping aid, she received proper medical treatment for her bipolar disorder.

It is important to remember that insomnia is usually a symptom of an underlying disorder or the manifestation of an illness. Examples of this are infection, chronic pain, stress, anxiety, metabolic or hormonal imbalance. The underlying disorders are often masked by prescription sleep aids. Taking a sleeping aid without trying to find out the reason for the sleep disorder can be dangerous.

I frequently see patients like Joan. She is starting to regularly have restless nights, and occasionally it is hard for her to fall asleep. She wakes up exhausted and then has an energy dip in the afternoon. She would like to exercise, but has no stamina or motivation.

When hormones start declining with age, sleep issues are common. Sometimes an illness or stressful situation can rob you of a good night's sleep. Whatever the underlying cause, if you are not getting adequate quality or quantity of sleep, then the release of hormones during sleep that regulate metabolism, appetite, and other key bodily functions will be impaired. If you have interrupted sleep, you will not make enough growth hormone, and your other hormones will be imbalanced.

They don't call it "beauty sleep" for nothing. Quality sleep helps your hormones to function optimally. With poor sleep, you're not going to feel that well, and you're not going to look that well either. In my practice, it's common for patients to complain of fatigue. And when I talk with them, I realize that they're not getting optimal sleep. It becomes a vicious cycle—not getting proper sleep, not having energy during the day, and then having difficulty sleeping. Balanced hormones help people to sleep, which generally will restore energy and stamina.

Poor sleep has other health consequences. It can increase the risk of heart disease.[3] Also, an alarming number of traffic accidents are related to fatigue, and there are studies showing that when people drive sleepy, they have the same impairment as people who drive drunk.[4]

The human body has a circadian rhythm, which is a 24-hour cycle that determines our sleeping and feeding patterns. It also affects brain wave activity and hormone production. When this circadian rhythm is interrupted, as it is for those who do shift work, that can cause problems in the circadian rhythm which can result in a shorter life span.[5] People who always do the night shift may not be producing optimal hormones.

I've cured insomnia in both women and men with hormone balance. Ed B. had issues with insomnia and migraines since puberty. He was in his early 40s when I saw him, and he said that for 30 years he had never been able to sleep well, and he had regular migraine headaches. After I optimized his testosterone level, Ed was able to sleep like a baby—for the first time since he was a teenager. His migraines also went away. Optimal testosterone levels in men, and optimal progesterone levels in women, help with quality sleep.

Cathy T., a retired sheriff, came to my office to refill her Ambien. She had been on Ambien for over 15 years and couldn't sleep without it. I asked her when she first noticed her insomnia. She exclaimed, "It came with those darn hot flashes." She said no other doctor had ever investigated why she was taking Ambien; they just kept refilling at her request. I prescribed Cathy bioidentical progesterone treatment, and after only one week she did not need to take another Ambien. She thanked me profusely for figuring out the underlying cause of her insomnia, and was so happy that I did not reflexively refill her prescription.

There are two types of insomnia. Traditional insomnia is difficulty falling asleep; then there's middle insomnia, which means you can fall asleep, but you wake up in the middle of the night. Some people have both types of insomnia. If you have issues with either type of insomnia, make sure that you visit your doctor and have things checked out, because it could be a sign that you have some kind of illness or an imbalance in your hormones. Sleep problems are something you need to fix, because fixing your sleep fixes so many other things in your body.

If everything checks out medically, then the next step, rather than going to a prescription drug, is to practice good sleep hygiene. That means having a routine that you follow when you are preparing to go to bed.

1) First of all, try to put yourself in a state of quietude, as we spoke about earlier; you want to relax, and get your mind and body still. Some people do this by taking a warm bath, or by meditating, stretching, or reading—whatever works for you and whatever you can do to quiet your mind and body.

2) Watching television or reading from a backlit screen tends to stimulate your brain, which then makes it hard for you to reach a state of quietude. It's recommended to turn off all electronics

about an hour before going to sleep, unless it's soft music or something relaxing.

3) For some people it helps to drink something warm, like chamomile tea. Tea with lavender or valerian root can also help people sleep. Or it could be hot chocolate—whatever is relaxing to you, and make sure it's caffeine-free.

4) Go to bed sleepy. If you're not sleepy, don't lie in bed hoping you're going to fall asleep. There are only two things that should take place in bed—sleep and sex. If you're not doing one of those two things, then get out of bed. You want your body to relate the bed with sleep. One of the best sleeping aids is to remove the television from your bedroom.

5) Make sure the environment is comfortable for you— that it's not too cold or too warm, that you have appropriate blankets, a good mattress, and the right pillow. If you have a history of allergies, invest in a hypoallergenic cover for your pillow and mattress.

6) Lastly, make sure that there is no light in the room, including light from electronics or phones. Charge all your electronics outside of your bedroom, and cover any lights coming from computers, television, or even the alarm clock—turn it to face it the other way. When there is no light entering your eyes, your brain is more likely to produce melatonin, which is the hormone that helps your body sleep.

ACTION:

CREATE YOUR OWN SLEEP HYGIENE ROUTINE

Think about your pre-bedtime practices. What elements can be added to your routine to better prepare your body for sleep?

NOTES:

1. Dement, William C., and Christopher Vaughan. *The Promise of Sleep: A pioneer in sleep medicine explores the vital connection between health, happiness, and a good night's sleep.* Dell Publishing Co, 1999.
http://psycnet.apa.org/psycinfo/2000-07284-000

2. Kripke, Daniel F., Lawrence Garfinkel, Deborah L. Wingard, Melville R. Klauber, and Matthew R. Marler. "Mortality associated with sleep duration and insomnia." *Archives of General Psychiatry* 59, no. 2 (2002): 131–136.
http://archpsyc.jamanetwork.com/article.aspx?articleid=206050

3. Laugsand, Lars E., Linn B. Strand, Carl Platou, Lars J. Vatten, and Imre Janszky. "Insomnia and the risk of incident heart failure: a population study." *European Heart Journal* (2013): eht019.
http://eurheartj.oxfordjournals.org/content/early/2013/02/28/eurheartj.eht019.abstract?sid=286f90b6/02ae/44dd/a9bc/8e84c04fb80e

4. http://drowsydriving.org/about/facts-and-stats/

5. Pati, Atanu Kumar, Arti Chandrawanshi, and Alain Reinberg. "Shift work: Consequences and management." *Current Science* 81, no. 1 (2001): 32–52.
http://www.iisc.ernet.in/~currsci/jul102001/32.pdf

R

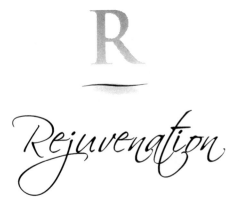

Rejuvenation

"*We don't stop playing because we grow old.*
We grow old because we stop playing."
—George Bernard Shaw

There are two aspects of rejuvenation I'd like to talk about. One is the rejuvenation of the mind, spirit, and soul; the other is the rejuvenation of the body. Let's first talk about mental and spiritual rejuvenation—achieved through relaxation and, yes, vacation.

The old adage about "working hard and playing hard" is often said in jest, but there's a lot of truth there. It's important to carve out time for yourself. It makes it possible for you to work more effectively and to take better care of others in your life. Personally, I know that I am a better doctor when I have taken better care of myself.

Caring for yourself and giving yourself time to rejuvenate mentally can begin with taking just five or ten minutes a day to rejuvenate. Listen to your body when it tells you that you need a break. It could be as simple as standing up and stretching, walking outside for a few minutes, or meditating for a few minutes.

When you are consciously thinking about things that you enjoy doing, you start anticipating them, and it restores a sense of youthfulness. Vacations are healthy! People hesitate to plan a vacation because of the cost or the time or because it is just not a priority. If extended and faraway vacations seem overwhelming, you can at least plan a day off or a long weekend. Or even a staycation. Do whatever is relaxing and enjoyable, and spend time with the people who bring you joy. You may decide you need some time alone to reflect and recharge.

I have a very fond memory of the time when my large extended family, about 50 of us, took a cruise together. It was a very nice way to spend time catching up with a huge group, because things are set up so that you don't have to worry about where you're going to eat or where you're going to meet. If people want to join you, they do. You don't have to plan heavily—you just have to get everybody on the ship. It was so great to rejuvenate with the family that means so much to me, many of whom I don't get to see that often because they live in a different part of the state. Having a reconnection or reunion like that recharges and rejuvenates the soul.

While sometimes my parents and in-laws complain that they don't have as much energy as they used to, I can see how much they enjoy being around children, and how it makes them more lively and energetic. I feel blessed to have my parents still around, and my in-laws as well, and they're so happy to have the grandkids around them. They say that the grandkids help keep them younger.

Sometimes you need a vacation or time away just with your partner. My husband and I plan an annual family vacation and then try to plan time for just the two of us. Even if it's just for the weekend. If the weekend doesn't work, at least do date night. It's important for couples to keep that connection and spend time enjoying each other. I felt guilty the first time I left my firstborn to have an "adult vacation." I called the house every day to check on him, and I could hear my son laughing in the background, enjoying time with his grandparents.

Instead of thinking that I was spending time away from my son, I started to think about it as time that he was spending with extended family members who love him. As the years passed, it became easier to leave the kids to have alone time with my husband. I will never forget the day I was explaining to my daughter about leaving for vacation. She was only four years old at the time, but she could see that I was concerned about leaving her. My daughter put her little hand on my heart and said, "Don't worry, Mama. I am always with you. You live in my heart." What four-year-old says that? Of course, I cried and it was hard to leave. At that point I realized how insightful and resilient kids are.

We have reviewed sleep and hormone imbalance in earlier chapters, and those are important factors in rejuvenation. Let's discuss some other relevant topics regarding rejuvenation.

For thousands of years the myth of the "fountain of youth" has been discussed, and even pursued by adventurers and explorers. To me, the fountain of youth is a symbol, a metaphor, of the power of water and its rejuvenation properties. The benefits of drinking sufficient water are numerous, as two-thirds of our bodies are made up of water. It's important to keep hydrated in order to keep our bodies in good working condition. When you don't drink enough water, many parts of your body suffer, the most visible being your skin. Skin gets drier when the body is not well hydrated, and dry skin enhances the appearance of wrinkles. The best way to moisturize dry skin is from the inside out, by drinking plenty of water. The water doesn't get rid of wrinkles, but it restores skin to a more supple state and helps minimize the appearance of wrinkles.

The Mayo Clinic recommends drinking eight glasses of water a day. For some people that might seem unattainable. Here's an example of a routine to get enough water: Drink a glass of water when you wake up, a glass sometime before and after each meal, and a glass an hour or two before bed. If you have issues with waking up at night to use the bathroom, it is better to have water at least two or more hours prior to bedtime. If you have issues with weight, drinking a glass of water before you eat will help to decrease your appetite. And if you work out, you may need to drink more water.

As we get older, we experience wear and tear on our joints. It's very common for people to start having osteoarthritic changes after age 40. The knees and hips are some of the most common deteriorations, and what that means is decreased mobility, decreased function, and less independence. In order to maintain our independence as we age, we need to do what we can to keep our joints healthy. It's important to keep our ligaments and tendons healthy as well.

One of the treatments I use with my patients to rejuvenate aging or injured joints is PRP (platelet-rich plasma) therapy. When you get a cut on your skin, the platelets help form a clot in the blood and help your skin to heal. PRP uses the patient's concentrated blood, which has high levels of platelets, and are integral for the healing process. Platelets contain growth factors that can stimulate soft tissue repair and regeneration. The growth factors help with the development of new blood vessels and aid in the wound healing process. When we administer PRP therapy, we take the patient's own blood and spin it down in a special centrifuge (we use the Harvest brand developed at Harvard University), then we inject the concentration of platelet-rich plasma directly back into the joints, such as the knees or shoulders.[1]

PRP works best on younger joints that are injured, usually from sport activities. As we get older, the spaces between the joints narrow due to the breakdown of cartilage or meniscus. PRP therapy helps to heal tendon and ligament injuries. Knee joints frequently lose space as we get older. Once the space in the knee joint is narrowed, sometimes to the point of bone on bone, then the damaged knees may need to be totally replaced with hardware. That surgery in itself can be very risky. PRP injections early on may delay the process of a total knee replacement. Also, PRP is a great alternative to cortisone injections. A study on arthritis showed that participants who took platelet-rich plasma had better functionality and less pain at the end of the study. It increased their mobility, which is key to longevity.[2]

I was featured on "The Doctors" in Spring 2014 with my patient who had severe cystic acne and hair loss. She had seen endocrinologists and dermatologists for her acne and hair loss and was offered birth control pills, spironolactone, and Rogaine. Her symptoms were getting worse, despite the prescription drugs. She was 30 years old and she was desperate for another option. Her hormone evaluation showed that she was low in progesterone and had estrogen dominance. She was elated when her skin cleared up and her hair grew back in a period of months after treatment of her hormone imbalance.

Her story inspired my patient Karen T. Karen is a 36-year-old African American woman who has been fighting hair loss since her early 20s. She is used to pulling her hair back tightly, close to her head, in a ponytail. She also used a special glue to keep a wig in place. She had hormonal imbalance and she suffered traumatic hair pulling due to her hair style. I started her on a hormone regimen, but she was anxious to have her hair grow back sooner. PRP therapy was used on her scalp to stimulate hair follicle growth. She was so excited to see hair growth just one month after the PRP injections. Besides improving her sleep and energy, the bioidentical hormones also helped her with hair growth.

Platelet-rich plasma therapy is also used for facial rejuvenation. It is marketed as a "vampire facelift." The PRP is injected directly into the face. It helps with collagen and elastin formation, improves skin texture and tone, and can be used to minimize wrinkle formation.

ACTION:

START REJUVENATING NOW!

If you aren't already drinking eight glasses of water a day, how can you increase your consumption of water?

What kind of break can you plan within the next six months—whether a vacation, a short mini-break, or a staycation? Schedule your next vacation or staycation this week.

Make a list of times when you can take daily breaks, and other little things you can do during your week that you enjoy and that will rejuvenate your body, mind, and spirit.

NOTES:

1. Kim, Dae Hun, Young Jin Je, Chang Deok Kim, Young Ho Lee, Young Joon Seo, Jeung Hoon Lee, and Young Lee. "Can platelet-rich plasma be used for skin rejuvenation? Evaluation of effects of platelet-rich plasma on human dermal fibroblast." *Annals of Dermatology* 23, no. 4 (2011): 424–431. **http://www.ncbi.nlm.nih.gov/pmc/articles/PMC3229934/**

2. Halpern, Brian, Salma Chaudhury, Scott A. Rodeo, Catherine Hayter, Eric Bogner, Hollis G. Potter, and Joseph Nguyen. "Clinical and MRI outcomes after platelet-rich plasma treatment for knee osteoarthritis." *Clinical Journal of Sport Medicine* 23, no. 3 (2013): 238–239. **http://www.ncbi.nlm.nih.gov/pubmed/23238250**

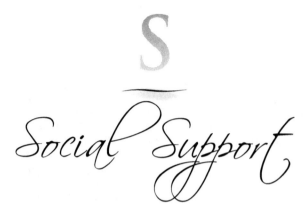

Social Support

"Love is our true destiny. We do not find the meaning of life by ourselves alone—we find it with another."

—Thomas Merton, *Love and Living*

Humans are social beings, and we need to have people around us who provide a network of caring social support. As we get older, this need becomes even more prominent. Having close relationships with people we love—a spouse, other family members, friends, or all of the above—is an important factor in health and longevity.[1,2]

Research has shown that having a permanent partner or spouse during midlife can reduce the risk of premature death.

The researchers in one study found that those who never married were more than twice as likely to die prematurely compared to those who had been in a stable marriage throughout their adult life.[3]

Unfortunately, there is a lot of loneliness among people at midlife and beyond. This loneliness is sometimes confused with depression, and doctors are likely to treat older people for depression without realizing that they might just be lonely. When somebody with loneliness gets treated for depression, one of the side effects of the medication can be apathy. The apathy can cause or contribute to depression. People don't feel like doing anything, which isolates them further and exacerbates the loneliness.

You may have heard about "Blue Zones," which are places in the world where people typically lead healthy lives until around 100 years of age.[4] There are five of these Blue Zones around the world, and one of the places is among the Seventh-Day Adventists in Loma Linda, California. The most well-known research has come out of Okinawa, Japan. After five years of researching the people who lived in the Blue Zones, it was affirmed that their lifestyle is what contributes to their longevity. They have a healthy diet, daily exercise, plenty of sleep, and a life that is low in stress. They have strong family ties, a sense of purpose, and spirituality is important in their lives. It's not surprising that such a lifestyle results in health and longevity.

What we can learn from life in the Blue Zones is that if we minimize stress and feel connected with the people around us, we will live longer and happier lives.

There's a great deal of research showing that stress has serious harmful effects on the body, mainly through the hormone cortisol, which is produced in high amounts during stress. When someone has a lot of either stress or anger in their life, their cortisol level is going to be increased, and this can have serious implications for blood pressure and heart disease.[5]

Studies have shown that social contact with close friends and relatives can reduce incidents of chronic disease, in particular cardiovascular heart disease, and delay mortality. One study highlighted that a feeling of loneliness was found to be associated with cardiovascular mortality, especially for males.[6]

There are also short-term health benefits to having a caring social network—notably that support from friends and family results in a reduced number of colds and flus. And people who have serious diseases actually recover quicker with social support.[7]

My husband's family is in central California, and although I don't see them often, I feel blessed to have their love in my life. Their kindness and strong family bonds are admirable. I was confident that my husband was going to treat me with care and kindness because I saw how much respect and love he had for his mom and sisters. I knew he would treat me well if he treated the important women in his life with respect and love. Our family get-togethers are filled with joy and appreciation for each other. Also, I am fortunate that my siblings and parents live in the same town as I do. I am so grateful for my 83-year-old father, who after walking three miles still has energy to pick up two of my kids from school. My parents lived in our home for 13 years and just recently moved into their own condo. My mom has been a continuous source of support in helping with my kids. We live the motto: "It takes a village."

Cultural expectations are different in various parts of the world. I was raised in the Filipino culture where aging family members are taken care of by their children or other relatives, and are not moved to a nursing home or live-in facility. All members of my family and extended family have always been taken care of by family members. Most commonly they will live in a daughter or son's home.

I have a fond memory of a 104-year-old patient—Nora W. She always came to see me with her 80-year-old daughter, and sometimes her 58-year-old granddaughter would come along. It was always good to see the three of them. Nora at 104 was still vibrant and going strong. She always came to the doctor's office with her hair done nicely and wearing a pretty outfit. Nora said she always wanted to look her best when she visited me because that would be her social event for the day.

It was wonderful to see that Nora had such strong family support. She never went to the doctor without a family member, and I could tell that the social connection, the bond that she felt with her family, was a strong source of support. The last time I treated her, which was for pneumonia, I could see that the care that her daughter provided was crucial in helping her to not only survive but recover more quickly.

As you age, keep in mind the importance of your social connections and your ties with those you love and care about.

I am a member of a Philippine American women's service organization called "Silayan Filipina."[8] It's a sisterhood that is built on networking and support between women from different professions and across the age spectrum. It provides Filipina role models who serve the community and empower youth through mentorship. We are connected by the values that we share and the community we serve. It is meaningful to me to be able to serve the community while cultivating our Filipino heritage. The friends and connections I have made are lifelong. I appreciate the mentorship, guidance, and support I have received from this group of women. Thank you so much, Joy, for reuniting our sisterhood.

I am so grateful for the women in my life that offer me even more than companionship; they are a source of love and support. I think of my friendships as flowers in a beautiful garden. Flowers need to be cared for—watered and nurtured. If the garden is neglected, the flowers will wilt and die. Have you seen a flower revive after you water it? Or noticed a flower open up when the sun comes out? I try to tend to my "garden," pulling out weeds so that the flowers can thrive. I can't imagine what my life would be like without my dear friends who are my cheerleaders and confidantes. Thank you Joann, Hollie, Connie, Michelle, Christie, Carol, Jen, Maria, Sherry, Alicia, Vickie, Lorena, Eva, Sonya, Luzvie, Karen, Eileen, Noeva, Mia, Sahlee, Sarah, Sheila and Rosanna for being the beautiful flowers in my garden.

Be mindful of the people in your life and community who are older than you, who might need just as much or more social support. Surround yourself with family and friends who share your interests and can support you. Do whatever you can to reduce stress in your life, making it more meaningful and happy.

ACTION:

CONTACT AND CONNECT

Strengthen the connection that you have with an older friend or relative in your life. Pick up the phone and have a conversation. Plan how you can spend some time together in person.

Notes:

1. Eisenberger, Naomi I., and Steve W. Cole. "Social neuroscience and health: neurophysiological mechanisms linking social ties with physical health." *Nature Neuroscience* 15, no. 5 (2012): 669–674.
http://www.nature.com/neuro/journal/v15/n5/abs/nn.3086.html

2. Wellman, Barry, and Scot Wortley. "Different strokes from different folks: Community ties and social support." *American Journal of Sociology* 96, no. 3 (1990): 558–588.
http://www.jstor.org/discover/10.2307/2781064?uid=3739560&uid=2&uid= 4&uid=3739256&sid=21104491019687

3. Siegler, Ilene C., Beverly H. Brummett, Peter Martin, and Michael J. Helms. "Consistency and Timing of Marital Transitions and Survival During Midlife: the Role of Personality and Health Risk Behaviors." *Annals of Behavioral Medicine* 45, no. 3 (2013): 338–347.
http://link.springer.com/article/10.1007/s12160-012-9457-3#page-1

4. Buettner, Dan. *The Blue Zones: 9 Lessons for Living Longer from the People Who've Lived the Longest.* National Geographic Books, 2012.
http://books.google.com/books?hl=en&lr=&id=fhJAn7fPkqAC&oi=f nd&pg=PR9&dq=blue+zones&ots=XMaq7lt2Va&sig=0XysPSSFGIP-GGe24gL6MqyMNel#v=onepage&q=blue%20zones&f=false

5. Bergland, Christopher. "Cortisol: why 'the stress hormone' is public enemy no. 1." *Psychology Today* (2013).
http://www.psychologytoday.com/blog/the-athletes-way/201301/cortisol-why-the-stress-hormone-is-public-enemy-no-1

6. Olsen, Rolf Bang, Jørn Olsen, Finn Gunner-Svensson, and Bodil Waldstrøm. "Social networks and longevity. A 14 year follow-up study among elderly in Denmark." *Social Science & Medicine* 33, no. 10 (1991): 1189–1195.
http://ideas.repec.org/a/eee/socmed/v33y1991i10p1189-1195.html

7. Clark, Corey M. "Relations between Social Support and Physical Health." (2007).
http://www.personalityresearch.org/papers/clark.html

8. http://www.silayanfilipina.com/

T
Trust Yourself

"Our deepest fear is not that we are inadequate. Our deepest fear is that we are powerful beyond measure. It is our light, not our darkness that most frightens us. We are all meant to shine, as children do. And as we let our own light shine, we unconsciously give other people permission to do the same. As we are liberated from our own fear, our presence automatically liberates others."

—Marianne Williamson

When you're making a decision, there's a certain visceral reaction—a gut feeling—that gives you a nudge about whether something is or isn't the right thing to do. Then sometimes you look at things from the perspective of your heart, meaning emotions are involved, which might not be the most objective. Other times you make decisions very objectively.

I think it's important to trust your instinct. Obviously, if it's a difficult decision, you also want to think objectively and evaluate the pros and cons. When the time comes to act, if you feel in your gut that you should go for something—or avoid something—experience has taught me to follow this intuition. From that point on, you have to trust that however you feel about the situation, and whatever reservations you have, you've made a commitment and you're going to go through with it. That's trusting yourself.

Many people either don't start toward a goal, or accomplish a goal, because they don't trust themselves, and so they don't commit. They let themselves down. A lot of it has to do with self-worth—or rather a lack of self-worth—which can be a result of previous failures, or, perhaps more often, based on what other people have said. I love the quote from Eleanor Roosevelt, "No one can make you feel inferior without your consent."

One time, I don't remember the exact circumstances, but my daughter said, "Mama, I'm afraid to do this. I don't think I'm good enough." I asked her, "Why do you think that? Who told you that you're not good enough?" And she said, "Well, my friend said it was stupid." I told her that when someone tells her something like that, it is not true unless she believes it.

Often people have a misconstrued negative idea about their own self-worth which does not come from within themselves, but from someone else. It might be someone who doesn't even know them that well—perhaps someone intimidated by their success, or who has no clue what they're going through. The point is, when you feel bad about yourself, when you feel you're not good enough, that's something that you allow yourself to feel. You don't have to allow that. It's not true unless you believe it. You can learn to trust yourself. There's a difference between a gut instinct, a deep sense of knowing what we are or aren't capable of, and holding back and not going for something because we're insecure and worried about what other people have said or will think.

There have been times when I had opportunities to start a business relationship with friends, but I didn't trust myself enough about the financial aspects; and in some cases I trusted friends too much. Part of it was not wanting to disappoint them, or let them down, or make them think I didn't have faith in them. If you ever have that gut instinct, that sense that something just doesn't feel right, I think it's important to pause and look at it more closely, without worrying about how the other person might react. If there's something that you honestly either feel concerned about or confident about, place more faith in yourself and your instinct than you do in the perceptions of others. And trust the right people.

I am very happy that I followed my instinct with the beverage business that my best friend and I co-founded. A lot of times people have a great idea, but don't follow through with it—and then someone else does and succeeds. I had that experience, and it was so frustrating.

When I was a freshman in medical school, I was traveling with my husband to San Felipe in Mexico in his 1969 VW bug. It was summer, and the car didn't have air conditioning, and it was so hot! I had a handful of vitamins in one hand and a water bottle in the other, and I thought, *I wish I could just drink my vitamins.* My throat was so dry, and I couldn't imagine swallowing all those pills. I told my husband what I was thinking, and he said, "That's a great idea, but how are you going to be able to do that?" And just that seed of doubt was enough for me to dismiss the idea, even though he didn't say it negatively.

Years later, when I saw water with vitamins at Costco, I actually kicked the crate. That was *my* idea! What made me even more upset was that this "water with vitamins" had sugar as a top ingredient and did not have therapeutic amounts of vitamins. The "vitamins" were a marketing tool—a good one, mind you. But if I was going to create something like that, I wanted a therapeutic amount of vitamins that would make a difference. A few years after that, I was telling this story to my dear friend and neighbor Connie Wesson, who is a successful businessperson and entrepreneur. She said, "If you want to make that kind of water, we can do it—and we can do it better." I asked myself if it was the right thing to do, and I got that tingle in my stomach and I realized that yes, it *was* what I wanted to do. Connie had the business sense and experience to help make it happen. I learned that besides trusting yourself, talking to and working with the right person makes a huge difference as to whether or not you go through with projects or goals. I knew in my heart, and gut, that I could trust Connie.

I was already in the field of anti-aging medicine, and Connie asked me, "What supplement do you think would be great to add to the water?" We thought about it and researched it, and we came up with resveratrol. There are a number of studies, some still in progress, regarding the benefits of resveratrol. Some of those benefits include decreasing the risk of diabetes by improving insulin sensitivity; helping maintain healthy weight and decreasing obesity; and perhaps most outstanding, cardioprotective effects. What a great supplement to bottle![1,2]

We set out to add resveratrol to water, and after two years of hard work and making sure we had the finest ingredients, we had developed Age Defense Water! I'm so proud of it, because we were true to our values and didn't compromise our integrity. There were three things I wanted our water to be: healthy, tasty, and affordable. Since energy drinks were in demand, we developed a healthy energy water with important supplements.

I felt lucky to partner with somebody that I trust as much as I trust myself. When you go into a business relationship with somebody, it's much like a marriage—you have to have the same values in order for it to work. Our company has succeeded because we share the same values, and we trust each other. We've already won design awards from *Beverage World* magazine. We started in a local store, one of the flagship Sprouts in south San Diego. We proved ourselves with consistent sales and, as a result, in spring 2014 we were in all 170 Sprouts. By fall 2014 we will be sold at Bristol Farms and Gelson's Markets, and we are looking to grow further.

Age Defense Water provides healthy energy, which can be helpful as we age, because we tire more easily. I wanted it to be healthy, and not to have any ingredients that were harmful, so we made it all natural—no sugar, no food dyes. It's sweetened with monk fruit and stevia and colored with vegetables. It not only contains resveratrol, but it's packed with other supplements as well, including ECGC (a polyphenol found in green tea) which has a positive effect on cardiovascular and metabolic health.[3] Each bottle has just five calories.

Caloric restriction has been shown to reduce your risk of diabetes and cardiovascular problems.[4] A 25-year study on caloric restriction published in *Nature Communications* in 2014 showed that monkeys who were not on a caloric-restricted diet had a threefold increased risk of death.[5] Other research showed that what we eat is also an important marker. It is not just about the absolute calorie count. Healthy diets in moderation were also shown to promote longevity.[6]

A scientific study showed that mice that took resveratrol, despite being on a high-calorie diet, had benefits that mimicked the benefits of caloric restriction.[7] Resveratrol has also been shown to affect the length of telomeres, which we talked about earlier in the chapter on Kindness. Longer telomeres mean decreased DNA damage and increased longevity.[8]

There are two forms of resveratrol—one is cis-resveratrol, the other is trans-resveratrol. Our water has trans-resveratrol, which is the active form that is metabolized by your body. Trans-resveratrol is found in foods like the skin of red grapes, which is why it is postulated that red wine is good for you. Red wine is believed to have cardioprotective effects, due to resveratrol.[9]

Age Defense Water can be found at Sprouts and Bristol Farms, and is due to appear in Gelson's Market in 2014. It can also be ordered online from our website: www.agedefensewater.com.

ACTION:

JOURNAL ABOUT TRUSTING YOURSELF

Were there times when you did not trust yourself or your gut instinct?

What were the results?

Do you have regrets about the decisions you made—personally or professionally—at those times?

Was there a time when you trusted yourself and something positive came of it?

NOTES:

1. You can find out more about Age Defense Water, as well as read a clear layman's explanation regarding the benefits of resveratrol, here: **http:// agedefensewater.com/about01.html**

2. Crandall, Jill P., Valerie Oram, Georgeta Trandafirescu, Migdalia Reid, Preeti Kishore, Meredith Hawkins, Hillel W. Cohen, and Nir Barzilai. "Pilot study of resveratrol in older adults with impaired glucose tolerance." *The Journals of Gerontology Series A: Biological Sciences and Medical Sciences* (2012): glr235. **http://biomedgerontology.oxfordjournals.org/content/early/2012/01/04/ gerona.glr235.short**

3. Wolfram, Swen. "Effects of green tea and EGCG on cardiovascular and metabolic health." Journal of the American College of Nutrition 26, no. 4 (2007): 373S-388S. **http://www.ncbi.nlm.nih.gov/pubmed/17906191**

4. Heilbronn, Leonie K., and Eric Ravussin. "Calorie restriction and aging: review of the literature and implications for studies in humans." *The American Journal of Clinical Nutrition* 78, no. 3 (2003): 361–369. **http://ajcn.nutrition.org/content/78/3/361.long**

5. Colman, Ricki J., T. Mark Beasley, Joseph W. Kemnitz, Sterling C. Johnson, Richard Weindruch, and Rozalyn M. Anderson. "Caloric restriction reduces age-related and all-cause mortality in rhesus monkeys." *Nature Communications* 5 (2014). **http://www.nature.com/ncomms/2014/140401/ncomms4557/full/ ncomms4557.html**

6. **http://www.nih.gov/news/health/aug2012/nia-29.htm**

7. Mercken, Evi M., Bethany A. Carboneau, Susan M. Krzysik-Walker, and Rafael de Cabo. "Of mice and men: the benefits of caloric restriction, exercise, and mimetics." *Ageing Research Reviews* 11, no. 3 (2012): 390–398. **http://www.ncbi.nlm.nih.gov/pubmed/22210414**

8. Palacios, Jose A., Daniel Herranz, Maria Luigia De Bonis, Susana Velasco, Manuel Serrano, and Maria A. Blasco. "SIRT1 contributes to telomere maintenance and augments global homologous recombination." *The Journal of Cell Biology* 191, no. 7 (2010): 1299–1313. **http://jcb.rupress.org/content/191/7/1299.short**

9. Russo, M. A., et al. "Sirtuins and Resveratrol-Derived Compounds. A Model for Understanding the Beneficial Effects of the Mediterranean Diet." *Endocrine, Metabolic and Immune Disorders Drug Targets* (2014). **http://www.ncbi.nlm.nih.gov/pubmed/25008762**

U

Understanding and Forgiveness

"Resolve to be tender with the young, compassionate with the aged, sympathetic with the striving and tolerant with the weak and wrong. Sometime in your life, you will have been all of these."

—Unknown

One of my patients shared with me her experience of having been taken advantage of by a man she loved and trusted. It devastated her, both emotionally and financially, and wounds like that don't heal quickly—it's been a process. What I find particularly interesting about her story is how the thing that helped her heal was coming to a better understanding of *herself* and of *why* she has found herself in several relationships with men who disappointed and abandoned her.

She realized how far back it went—to having been abandoned by her father, who loved her but wasn't physically there, because he chose to make work his priority at the time. She realized that this experience, which she still hadn't healed from, was also holding her back from forgiving this man who had abandoned her. As she became more aware of her history and her patterns and what was behind her actions, that understanding led to self-forgiveness, because she could be compassionate with the part of herself that got her into this situation. Instead of berating herself for making such a bad decision and for making such a big mistake in being with this man, she was able to understand that she had made this decision from a very young, wounded part of herself. And when she could see that, and accept that about herself, then she was able to forgive herself. Forgiving the man might be some distance away, because these things take time, but she's on her way towards forgiveness.

To me, self-awareness and understanding yourself means accepting yourself for who you are—the good and the bad, including all of your strengths, weaknesses, desires, wishes, fears, success, and failures. It's coming to a realization of who you are, and understanding that who you are is a result of the experience that you have had so far in life, the people you've met, and the relationships that you have (or have had) with those people.

When you have that understanding of who you are, that increased awareness, it's like a light at the end of a tunnel. The light will lead you out of where you're at, out of the darkness where your spirit is stuck. The light makes it clear which direction to move in; but first, you have to be honest with yourself and come to terms with your vulnerabilities. That honest reflection and true understanding might show you things you do not want to hear or see or feel, but if you can look at them squarely and accept yourself, then you can move forward. When you stop putting energy into trying to make something what it's not—trying to not be a certain way, or not have a certain feeling—but instead accept the way something is, or how you feel about it, then you can use your energy to start moving forward.

The way I see it, self-forgiveness is preeminent, because you can't forgive others until you have forgiven yourself. You have to understand your own vulnerabilities. Once you're able to forgive yourself—maybe for a mistake you made, or whatever you felt or did that got you into the vulnerable situation to begin with—then you are able to forgive the person who hurt you.

The process of forgiving somebody is very liberating. It releases a lot of negative emotions, so that you're not holding on to them anymore, and they're not holding on to you and dragging you down. But when you don't forgive someone, it's like a hatred that grows inside of you and festers.

Robert Muller says, "To forgive is the highest, most beautiful form of love. In return, you'll receive untold peace and happiness." I think that is a beautiful and profound statement. Forgiveness is manifesting self-love, and letting go of whatever disappointment, bitterness, self-loathing, or even hatred you are putting upon yourself.

If there's one regret I have, it's not recognizing sooner how when I was in college, I was blinded by love for a person who was emotionally hurtful toward me. Thank God I learned from it and didn't let that happen again, but I let it go on as long as I did because I believed in first love being lasting and true. There was also the promise that things would be different. I am very optimistic and give people the benefit of the doubt, and so I hoped things would be different, that it would be okay. When things didn't change, I blamed myself, as if it was my fault. It was a while before I could forgive myself for staying in the relationship so long. I couldn't move forward until I forgave myself, until I told myself and believed, "It is okay that I made a mistake and it was not my fault." It's not adversity that defines you. It's how you deal with adversity that determines your character. I tell my children, "People may take advantage of you and hurt you. Those people are your teachers; they teach you how to be resilient and patient. They teach you to be better."

It's not uncommon for women to make bad decisions in connection with their love for someone—and then, to blame themselves for those bad decisions. Part of it is a self-worth or self-respect issue. You blame yourself for being in a situation— as if you could have done something different to change that person's actions toward you, when usually that's not the case. A lot of women want to give their partner the benefit of the doubt, or give them another chance. The hope that something is going to change keeps them in that relationship; but when someone is hurtful, or selfish, or really doesn't care about you, all the hope in the world doesn't change that—unless they're willing to make the changes that they need to make.

One of the reasons to come to understanding and self-forgiveness, as well as to forgive others, is for the sake of your health and longevity. The more years you live, the more mistakes you are bound to make—and so as you age you have more opportunities, and more of a need, to forgive yourself and other people.

There is interesting research showing both the benefits of forgiveness and the consequences of unforgiveness. In one study there was a correlation between someone's ability to forgive and positive psychological traits such as self-esteem and satisfaction with your life. In the study, forgiveness was associated with positive emotional states, and MRIs showed that there were actually changes in the neural networks of the brain as a result of forgiveness.[1]

There was also a study that associated unforgiveness with declines in self-reported physical health.[2] Another study, specifically focusing on those aged 67 and above, showed that self-unforgiveness or unforgiveness by others had an indirect effect on depressive symptoms. If you have the ability to forgive, you're less likely to be depressed later in life.[3]

The moral of the story is, if you are hurt by somebody you care about, if you're able to come to an understanding of how and why it happened, to accept what's happened, to forgive yourself, and to forgive the person who wronged you, it will improve your quality of life. There is a good chance that in your lifetime you will be betrayed by a friend or lover, or someone will cheat you or lie to you. Each of us will face the challenge of forgiving and letting go. You can let go of anger and hostility, and experience positive emotions like high self-esteem and peace of mind. Forgiveness is both a coping mechanism and a healing mechanism. If we don't have the right coping mechanisms in place as we age, then that increases stress in our life, and we've already seen how stress causes ill effects to the body, and even kills. Extend understanding and forgiveness to yourself and others—it'll help keep you strong and reduce stress as you age.

ACTION:

FORGIVE YOURSELF

List three regrets that you have in life. In what way can you extend understanding and forgiveness toward yourself?

NOTES:

1. Ricciardi, Emiliano, Giuseppina Rota, Lorenzo Sani, Claudio Gentili, Anna Gaglianese, Mario Guazzelli, and Pietro Pietrini. "How the brain heals emotional wounds: the functional neuroanatomy of forgiveness." *Frontiers in Human Neuroscience* 7 (2013).
http://www.ncbi.nlm.nih.gov/pubmed/24367315

2. Seawell, Asani H., Loren L. Toussaint, and Alyssa CD Cheadle. "Prospective associations between unforgiveness and physical health and positive mediating mechanisms in a nationally representative sample of older adults." *Psychology & Health* 29, no. 4 (2014): 375–389.
http://www.tandfonline.com/doi/abs/10.1080/08870446.2013.856434#.U-roTeNdWSo

3. Ingersoll-Dayton, Berit, Cynthia Torges, and Neal Krause. "Unforgiveness, rumination, and depressive symptoms among older adults." *Aging & Mental Health* 14, no. 4 (2010): 439–449.
http://www.ncbi.nlm.nih.gov/pubmed/20455120

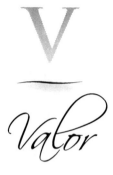

V

Valor

"*The ultimate measure of a man is not where he stands in moments of comfort and convenience, but where he stands at times of challenge and controversy.*"

—Martin Luther King, Jr.

Valor is courage, commitment, confidence, and action. It is believing in something, and then actually doing it. It's manifested in the actions you take when you are being your authentic self.

In order to be successful in life, we set out to fulfill our dreams and accomplish the things that we desire, but it takes more than just desire or even goals—it takes action! That action often requires courage, which translates to making a commitment to yourself. One of the things that motivates me is wanting to do the right thing. But sometimes it's easier to not do the right thing. It takes courage to be honest with myself, to know that the right thing might not be what everybody else is doing. It requires conviction to say, "I know that this is the right thing to do, and I'm going to do it because I'm committed to my belief."

As I see it, being courageous is staying on course, keeping the commitment you've made to yourself. It's very difficult. For most of my life, I have been in a position where I tried to please other people. Good or bad, that was my upbringing. I wanted to please other people, and that meant sometimes sacrificing my own desires, what I wanted for myself. I realized only later in life that this really wasn't serving anybody, because I wasn't being my authentic self with the people I loved. Instead, I was trying to figure out who they wanted me to be and trying to be that. That's just too complicated! Adapting yourself to other people results in betraying yourself. That's not good for your mental or physical health. We're not chameleons. The human spirit is unique in each of us, and if we can recognize that, and celebrate our differences, celebrate what makes us unique, then we can live our fullest life.

Not long ago I learned a special lesson about courage from a unique individual. I attended a diversity conference that highlighted taking care of LGBT (Lesbian, Gay, Bisexual, Transgender) patients. One of the speakers, a surgeon, shared his experiences as a transgender physician. Having been born male, he struggled most of his life knowing that his true gender identity was female. He was the epitome of the all-American male: he played football, joined the Navy, married a beautiful woman, and became a successful surgeon. To make a long story short, the time came when he felt so miserable about being trapped in a man's body that he confessed his gender identity to his wife. His wife supported his desire to be female. He later professed his gender identity to his colleagues and his patients. He continues to be a successful general surgeon, as a female. It did not seem to matter to most of his patients, because they admired his skill and expertise. I was touched by a poignant comment made by a fellow physician. He said, "If I allow *you* to be *you*, then it allows *me* to be *me*." If we can really be ourselves, then we can be truly successful in our endeavors.

Another kind of courage is maternal and paternal courage. I have seen a very moving example of this in Teresa, the daughter of one of my patients. Teresa got pregnant when she was 20 years old, and her baby's father left her because he didn't have the courage to make a commitment to either of them at that time. The baby, Elena, was born with hydrocephalus. At the time of birth, Elena underwent drastic surgery to have the fluid drained from her brain, and she survived. However, she can't see, she can't speak or communicate, and she can't move about or even sit up. In many ways she's like a living doll.

Teresa has completely dedicated her life to caring for Elena for the past 16 years. Being a parent is always challenging, and there are times for every parent when you feel your love and care for your child isn't reciprocated as fully as you'd like. But there are also times when their looks, their words and their hugs, validate everything and give us so much encouragement and warmth. Teresa has to go on without this, as Elena has never been able to tell Teresa that she loves her. But Teresa, with valor that I don't even know how to describe, continues caring for her daughter day in and day out—feeding her, bathing her, doing everything for her. She believes in the love that she and her daughter share, and showers Elena with the purest of unconditional love. I wonder if I would be capable of that kind of courage.

There's also emotional courage. How many people do you know who are afraid to make a commitment to a relationship, to another person? Many people desire to be in a meaningful and lasting relationship, but getting there requires commitment. It takes courage to get that relationship going, and to keep it going and growing. It takes making a commitment not only to the other person, but also to yourself—that you're going to be a loyal companion, a good listener, or whatever it means for you to be in a meaningful relationship. It takes courage to make that commitment.

Emotional courage is also the courage to keep going and move on when we've been betrayed by a lover, deceived by a friend, or cheated by a business partner. It's that courage that you muster up to say, "I need to move on and continue with my life." Sometimes you need to end a relationship, and it's hard to take a step that you know is going to give you short-term grief, even when you know it's going to be best for you in the long run. We don't like to suffer, but sometimes we'd rather suffer than make a courageous commitment or a courageous break. Many times people will choose not to rock the boat, to keep things as they are, because it takes too much courage and commitment to make the changes needed to make it better. You either suffer a little bit now, or you suffer a lot later. A person who has emotional courage decides that they'll suffer a little bit now.

A lot of steps toward wellness require emotional courage— things like exercising or changing your diet. In order to empower yourself to be healthier, sometimes you're going to need courage to make a positive change which takes effort, which takes commitment. It might be very hard. It might take a long time and a lot of "fight." Every day, all day, I have to talk to people about reducing their risk factors to certain diseases, which in many cases requires them to make difficult choices and commitments.

One of the most important factors in preventing disease is also one of the hardest things to give up—smoking! Tobacco use is the *number-one* preventable cause of disease, disability, and death in the United States.[1] It is a modifiable risk factor for some of the most serious and widespread diseases, such as heart disease and cancer. There was an article in *The New York Times* summarizing scientific research showing that nicotine is as addictive as heroin, cocaine, or amphetamines, and for most people, more addictive than alcohol.[2] In my many years practicing medicine and healthcare, I have seen more than enough evidence of this.

George S. was brought to my clinic in a wheelchair by his wife. His legs were amputated above his knees. He was a veteran, and I wondered if he had lost his legs in battle. He had, but it wasn't the battle I thought it was. He lost his legs to Buerger's disease, which is linked to smoking. In this disease, the blood vessels to the hands and feet get blocked, which can cause gangrene or infection, and if that progresses, can lead to amputation. People with Buerger's disease will tolerate amputation of body parts before they will quit smoking. This is a testament to the strength of tobacco addiction. George smoked until his legs were amputated to his thighs! Smoking can damage circulation and compromise blood flow starting at your extremities— the parts of your body furthest from your heart. Toes usually get compromised first. There was a study on veterans addicted to smoking in which they showed how their toes would be amputated, then their feet, then their legs, and some tolerated amputation all the way up to their thighs before they actually stopped smoking.[3,4]

The point is, it takes courage to make changes in lifestyle— especially when it requires giving up something we have grown attached to. It takes commitment, and that requires conviction, certainty, confidence, that you want to and are going to go through with it. Sadly, some people don't have the confidence that they're going to be successful. Their self-doubt, fear, lack of motivation, lack of confidence, holds them back.

As we go on this journey of life, at many points we pause and ponder what our next step will be, and need to summon courage to take that step. It might take everything we have in us to take that first step. It might be scary, there might be a lot of self-doubt, but that's part of the process. I am reminded of that quote, "A journey of a thousand miles begins with a single step." And it's okay to have missteps along the way; it's okay to even revise your journey along the way, but keep moving forward. Continue fulfilling that commitment to yourself with confidence and conviction. That is courage.

ACTION:

FACE YOUR FEARS

Are there challenges or fears keeping you from taking steps to improve your health? What are they? What changes would require courage? What are you really afraid of?

What is one thing you can do to be brave, to challenge your fear, and move into action?

NOTES:

1. http://www.cdc.gov/chronicdisease/resources/publications/aag/osh.htm

2. http://www.nytimes.com/1987/03/29/magazine/nicotine-harder-to-kickthan-heroin.html

3. Robinson-Whelen, Susan, and Carol Bodenheimer. "Health practices of veterans with unilateral lower limb-loss: Identifying correlates." *Journal of Rehabilitation Research and Development* 41, no. 3B (2004): 453–460. http://www.ncbi.nlm.nih.gov/pubmed/15543463

4. Bloom, R. J., C. A. Stevick, and S. Lennon. "Patient perspectives on smoking and peripheral vascular disease. A veteran population survey." *The American Surgeon* 56, no. 9 (1990): 535–539. http://europepmc.org/abstract/MED/2393193

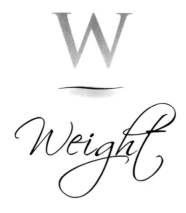

Weight

"*The older you get, the tougher it is to lose weight, because by then your body and your fat are really good friends.*"

—Unknown

One of the most rewarding aspects of my job is helping people become healthier by losing weight. It's a game changer. When people lose weight, it improves their sleep, energy, mood, sex, motivation, and stamina. It gives them the confidence to go for that job interview, or go out and look for a new partner. It boosts their self-esteem.

One of the reasons why I'm successful in helping people lose weight is that I convince people to do it for their health, and for longevity. I tell my patients, "Looking better is just a side effect of weight loss; it's not your goal. Good health is your goal, and health is beauty." When people are at a healthier weight, they feel and look better, and that helps their self-esteem. The end result is that they are healthier and happier.

Our society puts a lot of pressure on women to be thin. Unfortunately, I have seen the pressure begin at a very young age. I have seen it with my own daughter, who is thin as a rail. She can eat a healthy pasta dinner and then have post-dinner bloat and call herself fat! My daughter is very active and plays soccer. I like girls to be active in sports. When my daughter plays soccer, I want her to focus on the strength of her body, not how she looks in her soccer shorts. I want her to gain self-confidence because of her skill and talent.

One of the other soccer moms was upset because her daughter was sluggish on the soccer field, because she did not want to eat. When she asked her daughter why she did not want to eat, her daughter said, "My friend said I looked chubby, and asked me why I was gaining weight." We must keep in mind the power of our words and who is listening.

Parents sometimes bring their teenagers in to see me for weight loss. One of my favorite things to do as a doctor is to help adolescents lose weight. It not only changes their lives forever, it also changes the family dynamics. I stress to parents that in order for their children to eat healthfully, *they* have to eat healthfully. Who is buying the groceries? If you don't want your child to have soda at home, don't have it around as an option. Definitely easier said than done.

I will always remember Isabela. She was an honor student in high school, and active in sports. Her mother was very attentive to her diet, but it didn't seem to matter what Isabela ate, she was bloated—from her face to her feet. She saw many doctors and they were baffled by her progressive weight gain. Isabela did not eat sugar or gluten, and she exercised daily. You can imagine Isabela's frustration. Her mother bought her organic foods and would prepare all her meals and foods—even make her own trail mix for snack! It was so admirable how dedicated this mother was to making sure her family ate healthy, which only fueled her frustration about her daughter's weight gain. (As we will touch on later in this chapter, it is important to do an "emotional history" to discuss any psychological trauma. Fortunately, Isabela did not have any emotional trauma.)

I did an extensive evaluation of vitamin and mineral deficiencies, including comprehensive testing for any food intolerances. The results were surprising. Isabela was found to have intolerances to food that she thought was good for her. I discovered that she had leaky gut syndrome. We detoxified her gut, liver, and kidneys, and she avoided the foods she had intolerance to. Her mother was instrumental in helping her heal her gut using a special diet (which is beyond the scope of this book). Isabela was bloated due to inflammation, and once it was cleared from her system, she looked like a different person. No more spongy tissue around her neck and back. You could see the definition in her muscles. I was so proud and happy that she was able to start college with renewed self-confidence because she was healthier and happier.

When you focus on your health, and see weight loss as a part of that, you are removing the stigma and self-judgment regarding your outward appearance. It's not about how your body *looks*, it's about decreasing the fat around your organs inside your body, because *that's* what causes disease. One of the risk factors for heart disease is having too much fat around your belly, because that belly fat causes insulin resistance (which means your insulin is not as effective, and sugar can rise more readily in your blood, increasing your risk of diabetes).

In the days of hunters and gatherers, it was necessary for the body to hold on to fat, and it saved lives when people weren't sure that they were going to eat every day. That's why we call it the "spare tire." But nowadays, when we eat so much, often too much, we don't need that spare tire—but it's still there for us. On top of that, our metabolism slows down as we get older. We acquire more fat and lose lean muscle, so it's easier for us to gain weight. If you eat the same amount as you did last year, you will gain weight, because as you age, your body needs fewer calories to sustain life. There are some elegant studies that demonstrate how caloric restriction—decreasing the amount of calories that you eat on a given day—is one of the best things that you can do to promote longevity.[1]

You want the calories that you do consume to be nutritious, not empty. The goal is to nourish your body with food that your body knows how to process—whole foods. As we discussed earlier in the chapter on Detox, whole foods are available in a natural state—without refined sugars or preservatives, not processed and canned or wrapped in plastic. Some food for thought: Eat as fresh as possible. Look at ingredients and labels. If anything has more than four ingredients, and half of them are words you can't pronounce, some of them are most likely preservatives. Preservatives can make or keep you fat, so you want to limit your intake or not eat them.

To find your ideal weight, one of the most objective things that you can use is the Body Mass Index (BMI). I'll include a link at the end of this chapter to help you find yours. An ideal BMI is between 19 and 25. Above 25 is considered overweight. Above 30 is considered obese.

Bone size is a factor, so BMI is not 100% accurate for everyone. There are small, medium, and large body frames. If you have a large body frame, then your ideal BMI and weight will be higher.

To determine body frame size, you can measure the wrist with a tape measure and use the following list to determine whether a person is small, medium, or large boned.[2]

Women

Height under 5'2":

Small = wrist size less than 5.5"

Medium = wrist size 5.5" to 5.75"

Large = wrist size over 5.75"

Height 5'2" to 5'5":

Small = wrist size less than 6"

Medium = wrist size 6" to 6.25"

Large = wrist size over 6.25"

Height over 5'5":

Small = wrist size less than 6.25"

Medium = wrist size 6.25" to 6.5"

Large = wrist size over 6.5"

Men

Height over 5'5":

Small = wrist size 5.5" to 6.5"

Medium = wrist size 6.5" to 7.5"

Large = wrist size over 7.5"

BMI should be routinely checked for patients and is considered the fifth vital sign. The vital signs typically checked in a doctor visit are temperature, respiratory rate, heart rate, and blood pressure. It's an objective measurement that we can follow and monitor. When you take your kids to the pediatrician, they check height and weight and head circumference, and if a child is off the curve, it is a red flag to take action. Unfortunately, obesity is on the rise among the pediatric population. When I graduated from medical school in 1993, type 2 diabetes was called "adult-onset diabetes." Today we are seeing type 2 diabetes as early as adolescence. One of the best ways to prevent it is to prevent fat from accumulating around the belly.

I'd like to share some of the success stories of people whom I've helped to lose weight, including some letters from patients. (You can find before-and-after photos of some of my clients by going to my website: www.drmelindasilva.com.)

Kelly M. is a 34-year-old Caucasian female with type 2 diabetes. She originally visited my clinic for weight loss. She was on 28 different medications for her diabetes, high blood pressure, high cholesterol, chronic pain, anxiety, and depression. Unfortunately, her type 2 diabetes was difficult to control and her endocrinologist put her on an insulin pump.

I focused on lifestyle changes for Kelly. I balanced her hormones. I used the Human Chorionic Gonadotropin (HCG) diet as a tool to help her to lose weight. I use a modified version, rather than using the traditional HCG diet, and I only use it as a short-term tool. With the HCG diet, most women will lose 15 to 20 pounds in six weeks, and most men will lose 20 to 30 pounds. This diet has to be supervised by a doctor. The FDA does not approve it for weight loss and does not like the 500 calorie diet that has been associated with HCG since it began in the 1950s. I also do not approve of the 500 calorie diet. People should not buy the online versions of HCG because it may be harmful and it cannot be validated as being uncontaminated. HCG is a controlled substance and should only be administered by a doctor.

Kelly followed the HCG diet for six weeks, to give her a kick-start on her weight loss and motivate her. She was slipping into major depression, so it was really important to help her to lose weight quickly. At the end of two months she had lost 35 pounds, and she went from taking 28 medications to only taking 2 medications! I got her off all of her medications for anxiety and depression, chronic pain, and cholesterol. She had been on four medications for high blood pressure, and I reduced her to half a pill. She had been on four medications for diabetes, and now she only has to take the smallest dose of insulin possible.

Her HgbA1c had been at 14.8% (meaning average blood sugar at 378, which is really high). For those with diabetes, the goal is to have HgbA1c at less than 7% (average blood sugar at

154) to reduce the risk of diabetes complications. Despite Kelly being on four diabetes medications, her mainstream primary care doctor had only been able to get Kelly's HgbA1c down to 12% (average blood sugar at 300). After I balanced Kelly's hormones and helped her to lose weight, her HgbA1c went down to 4.8% (average blood sugar at 91). Her HgbA1c level was actually better than mine, and I don't have diabetes! Kelly told me that her primary care doctor said, "Whatever Dr. Silva's doing for you, keep doing it, because she's making me look good."

After the weight loss and mood changes were resolved, Kelly looked about 15 years younger, and most importantly, she was happy and felt stronger! She became functional, productive, able to take care of her family, and it saved her marriage. One of the best things that happened for Kelly's family is that because she lost weight and felt so good, she was able to motivate her obese teenage daughter to control her weight. When Kelly ate healthier, the whole family ate healthier. I was able to take care of Kelly's daughter as well, and it gave me great satisfaction to help her lose weight. Now she is going to have a better chance at good health, and may prevent diabetes. The weight loss and good health altered the dynamics of the family. That's what I mean about losing weight being a game changer.

Another of my favorite success stories is that of Paul Schatz. He was 65 when he came to see me, weighing over 300 pounds, and diagnosed with prediabetes and borderline hypertension. The fear of diabetes motivated him to get the help he needed to lose weight. I helped him lose over 105 pounds in one year, and the good news is that three years later, he's kept it off.

One of the things that really bothered him was tremendous knee pain; because he was so heavy, he could barely walk. Once he lost weight, he had less pain in his knees, which gave him more freedom and mobility, and that changed his life. He was no longer prediabetic. He didn't have to take any medicine for blood pressure. All of his labs, including cholesterol, were normal. After he lost 105 pounds, he brought in a pair of jeans that fit him at his heaviest weight and it looked like both he and I could have fit into his old jeans!

To help him lose 105 pounds, I put him on HCG and incorporated a whole food diet program. To maintain his weight, Paul has to maintain the lifestyle of choosing healthy whole foods and staying active. That is not to say that to live healthy and keep weight off you can't celebrate life with comfort food from time to time. Moderation is the key. The best thing about HCG is that it changes a person's relationship with food. HCG changes people's cravings, and when you're able to change people's cravings, then they're able to keep weight off. I require people to eat only whole foods with the HCG diet, and that forces them to acquire the healthy habit of eating whole foods.

When you consistently eat a food, your body will soon crave that food.

Paul was very successful at changing his lifestyle, and it motivated him to help others. He now actually wants to quit his job as an interior designer—and this is a gentleman whose success as a designer was featured in *The New York Times* recently. He has started a lifestyle coaching program called NutraGuia to help other people lose weight by teaching them how to eat well. He serves as a mentor and coach and offers tasty sustainable meal plans to maintain weight loss through NutraGuia.[3] The most important thing about Paul's work is that he educates and empowers patients to prepare healthy meals for themselves.

Sometimes it's not easy to help people lose weight. Gina W. was 340 pounds at her heaviest. She is 44 years old, and has been on every popular diet for the past 20 years. She has been successful at losing weight in the past, she just does not seem to be able to keep it off. After doing a medical history, I often do what I call an "emotional history" to try to get a better understanding of my patient. Gina's parents divorced when she was quite young, her mother died from a terrible drug overdose, and she was molested by her stepdad. Gina had a baby when she was 22 and ended up being a single mom. After her pregnancy, she could not lose the weight, and steadily gained more weight.

When I was practicing primary care, I learned that one of the most important indicators in someone's health is how they feel emotionally. Psychological factors and emotions have a huge impact on health, especially weight issues. In 2010, *Time* magazine reported on the results of a study by Dr. Vince Felitti from Kaiser San Diego which revealed that childhood trauma can cause adult obesity. The more adverse childhood experiences someone had, the more likely they would be obese. Sometimes overeating is a coping mechanism for anger, anxiety, or fear.[4] One of Dr. Felitti's patients said, "Overweight is overlooked. That's the way I need to be." It is important to remember that we should have our psychological needs addressed, as well as our physical needs, in order to reach our optimal health.

Here are two testimonials written by my patients:

Rebecca K.

I first met Dr. Silva about three months ago. I had been having problems with my thyroid for the last two years. During that time, I gained 25 pounds. I felt exhausted all the time, I couldn't sleep well, and I couldn't think clearly. As a teacher, I have to be on my feet for hours and have the energy to teach others. My poor health was having a terrible impact on my life.

I visited four different doctors in the U.S. and Mexico to get help. Each of them told me something different and two of them didn't even believe that

I had a problem. I had a miscarriage and started to feel more anxious and depressed. No one offered me a way to wellness. I was desperate and at the end of my rope. Then a good friend of mine recommended Dr. Silva.

At my first appointment, Dr. Silva spent over an hour with me listening to my medical history, reviewing my lab results, and discussing my options. I was impressed with her sincerity and genuine concern for my health. Dr. Silva prescribed a natural thyroid medicine for me, and it made a major difference. She also put me on a detoxification diet that led to me losing five pounds in ten days—something I hadn't been able to achieve with numerous diets and nearly starving myself. The detoxification diet also helped me to identify foods that weren't good for my body. In addition, I was prescribed a multi-vitamin regimen that has helped my energy levels tremendously.

I am nearing the end of a second specialized diet using HCG, and after just 40 days I reached my weight goal. I feel energized when I wake up in the morning, and I still have energy after work in the afternoons. I have clarity of mind at last, and I feel happy and healthy again. Meeting Dr. Silva helped me to regain my health and my positive outlook on life. I highly recommend her to anyone wishing to improve their well-being!

Mark P.

The HCG Diet, when administered by a licensed doctor, really works. The results are amazing!

I have been concerned about my weight for around 10 years, but never really had the time or willpower to do something about it. Recently I realized I was having a hard time keeping up with my kids, experiencing difficulty sleeping, and generally just felt out of energy. Worse than any of that, though, was the shock I received when I took my most recent family picture—I was huge!

The weight didn't come on all at once. Over the last decade, I have probably steadily put on about 5 pounds per year. While one year I took some initiative and lost about 25 pounds through vigorous workouts, it was a lifestyle that I couldn't sustain—hey, I was a college student, working more than one job, and once I found a new girlfriend (now my wife), I unfortunately chose to sacrifice my gym time to get everything else done. The weight came back and continued to climb. My BMI reached 34, and I knew that over 30 was considered obese. One of my doctors told me that it was time to start paying attention to my body's needs.

While I have been steady at around 250–255 lbs. for the past year or so and knew that I was overweight, I just couldn't seem to lose any weight by doing what I thought would really help—cutting and counting calories. My primary care physician told me to cut things like bread and focus more on vegetables. I ate a lot of veggies as instructed, but only lost 4 lbs. over the course of 8 months. This was too slow. I wanted to exercise, but my body would hurt so much after exercise, and I kept getting sick. I needed something that would kick-start my weight loss and help me "reset" my body. Then my wife learned about HCG and introduced me to it.

As it was explained to me, you take HCG, cut your calories, and minimize exercise while on HCG. By doing this, the claim was that I could lose 30–40 lbs. What?! This intrigued me, so I started to learn more about it. I found out that there are many strains of HCG out there, but only a couple that are the legitimate product, and to be safe, I wanted to have a doctor help me. I tried walking into a clinic that was offering the product at a reduced rate, but found it to be too far away and I wasn't sure if it was the real HCG or not. That's when I came across Dr. Melinda Silva. Her office was very helpful, and someone walked me through the process before I even set foot in the office. I knew what to expect every step of the way, which made the journey a lot smoother for me.

I started the HCG diet with a weight of 257.6 lbs. Forty days later, I stood on the scale and weighed 213.6 lbs.—44 lbs. lighter! I haven't been this thin since I was married. How do I know? The pants I bought around that time and quickly outgrew were the only pants that would fit me—all my other clothes were just too big! I had kept them in the closet as a "target" for some future date, and now I have arrived at that future. While I still have a few pounds to lose (my target is 170), I am well on my way!

The most amazing thing to me about the diet was that even though I felt hungry, I was not overwhelmingly hungry. I was able to follow the instructions to the letter and the weight just peeled off. I realized through the program that I needed to make a lifestyle change, and not just take off the weight temporarily. I invested in the program with money, time, and effort. I am now able to maintain and even continue to lose from that point, weighing in at 205.6 lbs. as I write this. I lost an additional 8 lbs. since I have been off HCG. I really believe that the program has allowed me to reset my hypothalamus, and the smarter choices I make now when I eat are paying off. Also, now that I am lighter I have less back pain and indigestion, more energy, less strain on my knees, and more confidence. I have another problem now—I have to buy a new wardrobe!

I really want to thank Dr. Silva and her staff for their incredible support with my transformation, and express my heartfelt gratitude for their guidance over the past few months. I am taking this opportunity to really change and make this stick!

A few things in closing: Reaching a healthy weight is life-changing and in many cases life-saving. Obesity can cut longevity by increasing your risk of heart disease, which is the number-one killer, along with increasing your risk of cancer and diabetes. I agree with the saying that "Diet is a four-letter word." What really makes a difference is focusing on having a healthy weight. Think about changing the way you eat for the rest of your life. Your relationship with food has to change. That's not to say that you can't have your favorite treat now and then. That's not to say that when you go on a vacation you can't eat the local cultural foods, or taste your favorite comfort foods once in a while. You can even allow yourself a cheat day once a week. It's about moderation. It's about making healthy choices normally on a daily basis. And when you make an unhealthy choice, or when you go on a vacation and gain that pound or two, you're aware of it, and do what you need to do to lose that weight. Regularly weighing yourself is important, because if you're cognizant of your weight, you're less likely to "let yourself go."

ACTION:

MEASURE, WEIGH, AND RECORD

Calculate your BMI. You can find out what it is here: http://www. nhlbi.nih.gov/health/educational/lose_wt/BMI/bmicalc.htm.

Weigh yourself naked every morning using a digital scale for one month, so that you can keep a close watch on how your body reacts to different foods.

Keep a food journal for a week. Or, if you can, for a month is better. Write the date, the time you eat, and list all food, including condiments and beverages. (You can also note in your food journal whether you exercised that day.)

NOTES:

1. Roth, George S., Donald K. Ingram, and Mark A. Lane. "Caloric restriction in primates and relevance to humans." *Annals of the New York Academy of Sciences* 928, no. 1 (2001): 305–315.
http://www.ncbi.nlm.nih.gov/pubmed/11795522

Masoro, Edward J. "Overview of caloric restriction and ageing." *Mechanisms of Ageing and Development* 126, no. 9 (2005): 913–922.
http://www.ncbi.nlm.nih.gov/pubmed/15885745

2. http://www.nlm.nih.gov/medlineplus/ency/imagepages/17182.htm

3. http://nutraguia.com/en/index.php

4. http://content.time.com/time/health/article/0,8599,1951240-1,00.html

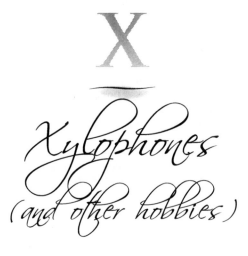

X

Xylophones
(and other hobbies)

"Today is life—the only life you are sure of. Make the most of today. Get interested in something. Shake yourself awake. Develop a hobby. Let the winds of enthusiasm sweep through you. Live today with gusto."

—Dale Carnegie

Hobbies are one of the pieces of the puzzle that contributes to life balance. It's healthy to have something to look forward to. We all get caught up in our work, thinking about all the things on our to-do list, and then we get home and have a second to-do list of the things we must do to take care of our families and our households. So having a hobby can be an escape from busyness, from responsibilities, and the chaotic things that happen in your life. It can also be a creative outlet, which some people need to balance them. It's fuel for your soul.

When we do things that engage our mind, things that are challenging or rewarding for us (or both), it helps us to be creative in our life in general. That means it also makes our work life better, and most of all, it makes for an increase in our quality of life. We have higher levels of satisfaction and happiness when we do something that we enjoy, so hobbies can enrich our lives. Remaining active and having leisure activities later in life contributes to healthy aging.

There's research from UCLA in the *Journal of Aging and Health* documenting the physical and psychological benefits of remaining active later in life, showing that exercise and participation in leisure activities are predictive of better perceived health and greater life satisfaction.[1]

Hobbies and creative interests can also help us expand our social circles. They are a good way to meet other people who have similar interests. Being socially active is important for the elderly. Sadly, there is a high rate of loneliness among the elderly, which can contribute to mental health issues, including suicide, and can increase the chance of mortality. In the *American Journal of Geriatric Psychiatry,* a study revealed the factors associated with attempted suicide in the elderly, and there was an association between perceived loneliness—usually among those unmarried and living alone—and attempted suicide.[2]

So having hobbies, doing things that are fun and interesting, helps you age better, and is also part of building the social support network that you need as you age.

My friend was telling me the other day about her 96-year-old neighbor who still lives in his own house. He's self-sufficient, independent, and has frequent visits with his friends. They come over and take him to casinos or on other outings a few times a week. They hang out at his place and play cards and board games. His daughter also visits him every day. He has an incredibly active social life, and it's fairly apparent that it contributes to his longevity. He's 96 and going strong.

One of my favorite hobbies right now is yoga. I didn't start yoga until I was 50 years old, and I wish I had started earlier. I can only imagine how much stronger I would be. I have had friends comment, "Wow, how do you stay so fit? You must exercise every day." I wish I did, but in reality, I practice yoga just once or twice a week. Truth be told, I exercised intensely in the beginning to get the body I wanted (with CrossFit, Pilates, yoga, cycling, etc.). Once you are where you want to be, it's much easier to keep yourself there with maintenance. It's when you let yourself go and don't do anything regular that it becomes difficult. That's why I can practice yoga once a week and maintain my tone. Yoga keeps my core strong, which keeps everything else strong. It helps me to feel relaxed. I think of yoga as meditation in action. I am the ultimate multitasker, and I joke with my friends about how I am multitasking with yoga because I can exercise and meditate at the same time!

There are many things I enjoy about yoga. I feel as if I can take deeper breaths, I like the way it has increased my flexibility, and my muscles feel less tight. After a long day at work I can stretch and do yoga, and it helps me relax. My neck muscles loosen up and my carpal tunnel symptoms seem to improve. There is an article in the *International Journal of Yoga Therapy* showing the psychological benefits of yoga practice for older adults,[3] and another study showed that yoga can assist with health challenges by alleviating everyday stress and decreasing anxiety and depression.[4] Stress and anxiety contribute heavily to chronic disease and decreased quality of life, and yoga can be used as non-pharmacologic therapy to help relieve stress and anxiety.[5,6] This is important for the older population, who may often be taking many pharmaceutical drugs.

One study of yoga and back pain showed that when premenopausal women with chronic low back pain practiced yoga three times a week for twelve weeks, back flexibility was improved and chronic low back pain improved.[7] Another study showed that intensive yoga reduced pain-related disability and improved spinal flexibility, which improved chronic low back pain. It was more effective than a regular physical exercise regimen.[8] All that to say, yoga can be a great hobby.

Whatever your hobby preference, the main point is to have one! Practice it, enjoy it, be active, and it'll help you age gracefully and strong.

ACTION:

PICK A HOBBY

List some hobbies that you enjoy. Don't forget about hobbies that you enjoyed when you were younger. Or pick new ones. Or a mixture of old and new.

Schedule time in the next week to participate in one of these hobbies on your list. Better yet, ask a friend to participate with you.

NOTES:

1. Menec, Verena H., and Judith G. Chipperfield. "Remaining active in later life: the role of locus of control in seniors' leisure activity participation, health, and life satisfaction." *Journal of Aging and Health* 9, no. 1 (1997): 105–125.
http://jah.sagepub.com/content/9/1/105.short

2. Wiktorsson, Stefan, Bo Runeson, Ingmar Skoog, Svante Östling, and Margda Waern. "Attempted suicide in the elderly: characteristics of suicide attempters 70 years and older and a general population comparison group." *The American Journal of Geriatric Psychiatry* 18, no. 1 (2010): 57–67.
http://europepmc.org/abstract/MED/20094019

3. Bonura, Kimberlee Bethany. "The psychological benefits of yoga practice for older adults: evidence and guidelines." *International Journal of Yoga Therapy* 21, no. 1 (2011): 129–142.
http://www.ncbi.nlm.nih.gov/pubmed/22398354

4. Li, Amber W., and C. A. Goldsmith. "The effects of yoga on anxiety and stress." *Alternative Medicine Review* 17, no. 1 (2012): 21–35.
http://www.ncbi.nlm.nih.gov/pubmed/22502620

5. Smith, Caroline, Heather Hancock, Jane Blake-Mortimer, and Kerena Eckert. "A randomised comparative trial of yoga and relaxation to reduce stress and anxiety." *Complementary Therapies in Medicine* 15, no. 2 (2007): 77–83.
http://www.ncbi.nlm.nih.gov/pubmed/17544857

6. Javnbakht, M., R. Hejazi Kenari, and Majid Ghasemi. "Effects of yoga on depression and anxiety of women." *Complementary Therapies in Clinical Practice* 15, no. 2 (2009): 102–104.
http://www.ctcpjournal.com/article/S1744-3881%2809%2900004-8/abstract

7. Lee, Moseon, Woongjoon Moon, and Jaehee Kim. "Effect of yoga on pain, brain-derived neurotrophic factor, and serotonin in premenopausal women with chronic low back pain." *Evidence-Based Complementary and Alternative Medicine* 2014 (2014).
http://www.ncbi.nlm.nih.gov/pubmed/25120574

8. Tekur, Padmini, Chametcha Singphow, Hongasandra Ramarao Nagendra, and Nagarathna Raghuram. "Effect of short-term intensive yoga program on pain, functional disability and spinal flexibility in chronic low back pain: a randomized control study." *The Journal of Alternative and Complementary Medicine* 14, no. 6 (2008): 637–644.
http://www.ncbi.nlm.nih.gov/pubmed/18673078

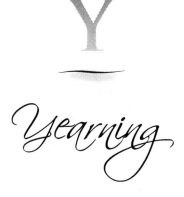

Y

Yearning

"*We are desire. It is the essence of the human soul, the secret of our existence. Absolutely nothing of human greatness is ever accomplished without it. Not a symphony has been written, a mountain climbed, an injustice fought, or a love sustained apart from desire. Desire fuels our search for the life we prize.*"

—John Eldredge

What do you desire most in life? What do you yearn for? I yearn to love. I yearn to serve. I yearn to connect. I yearn to be happy.

One thing that tops the list or makes the short list for most people is having meaningful relationships. This includes lasting friendships, a strong marriage, and social connections. We thrive on social interaction.

There was an interesting study reporting how social relationships can actually predict odds of survival, and that strong social connections with friends, families, colleagues, or neighbors can improve your odds of survival by 50 percent. The influence of social relationships on risk for mortality is comparable with well-established risk factors for mortality. For example, minimal social interaction has the same risk level as being an alcoholic. Minimal social interaction is more harmful than not exercising, twice as harmful as obesity, and equivalent to smoking 15 cigarettes a day. I find that impressive and amazing![1]

The researchers studied 148 published longitudinal studies on the subject of human interaction and related health outcomes, and reviewed the studies over a period of seven and a half years on average. It showed that there are many ways that friends and family influence health for the better, ranging from a calming touch to helping find meaning in life.

When someone feels socially connected to other people, they have a higher sense of purpose or meaning, and that translates to their desire to take better care of themselves, and take fewer risks, so that they can maintain or increase their social interaction with the people they care about. This study validates what I innately know to be true—that we all need each other at a very fundamental level. The bottom line is that people who are in meaningful relationships have better health and higher life expectancy.

"The Longevity Project,"[2] an eighty-year research study eventually published as a book, shows a clear connection between having a productive and meaningful life and long-term health. It busts some common myths. For example, people do not die from working long hours at a challenging job—many who worked the hardest actually lived the longest, which connects with what we looked at in the chapter on priorities and productivity. Longevity is not a result of purely physical causes—a matter of having proper diet and exercise and sleep and that's it. You also have to look at other components of life, and social interaction and a purposeful life are big factors. Connecting this back to desire—or yearning—if there is something you really want, something that adds meaning to your life, that you care about and work for, then that desire and the related productivity can contribute to your longevity.

Relationships factor in, and the research didn't show that being married automatically leads to a healthy, long life. The focus is on being in healthy and meaningful relationships, more so than just getting and staying married. The concept that married people had greater longevity was more applicable to men than women, and marriage was only health-promoting to the extent that it was a *good* marriage. So it's not about just being married, but feeling happy in that marriage or relationship. It's better to be single or divorced and happy than married and unhappy.

Sometimes we women are hesitant to speak about what we really desire, or even to admit it to ourselves—whether it's a desire for a relationship, for a change in a relationship, for intimacy, to pursue a project or business, or to engage in a hobby or activity that makes us happy. It's difficult for many women to actually feel okay about pursuing our desires, whatever they are.

In many cases we have become so conditioned to care for others that we put our own desires on the back burner, and sometimes we lose touch with them to the point that we don't even know what they are anymore. It's important that we connect with our own desires, that we allow ourselves the freedom to yearn for and pursue the things that we desire—it helps give us a sense of purpose and keeps us aging gracefully.

If you have become detached from your own desires, then developing a vision of how you want to see the rest of your life unfold is a very useful and inspiring thing. Creating a vision board can help provide clarity and give you a road map toward pursuing your desires and reaching your goals.

You might say "I want to be happier" or "I want a better life" or "I want a better relationship." But what do you really mean by that? Do you even know? A vision board, or journaling, can help you to get much more specific. What does that happiness feel like?

What does that better life look like? What does the relationship of your dreams involve?

Creating your vision board is part of the process of helping you to visualize your desire, which in turn will make it come true. When you create a vision board, you find symbols or pictures that help solidify or describe your desires or goals, or the feelings or experiences that you want to have.

As for how to create your vision board, a simple method often used is to look through magazines and find pictures of things that correspond to desires you have. When you find something, rip the page out of the magazine and cut out the image that reminds you of a desire that you have, or that you can associate with a desire that you have. Put several of those on a board. You might choose one particular desire, or you might choose a few desires or visions that you have. And that's the beginnings of a vision board. Have fun with it!

ACTION:

WHAT DO YOU YEARN FOR?

What are your desires in life? Are you doing what you need to do to fulfill your desires? If not, why not?

Create a vision board illustrating one or several of the things you desire.

If you could wave a magic wand and create the life of your dreams, and time or money were no object, what would your life be like?

* Who would you be?
* Who would you be with?
* What would you be doing?
* Where would you live?
* What would a day in your life be like?

Notes:

1. Holt-Lunstad, Julianne, Timothy B. Smith, and J. Bradley Layton. "Social relationships and mortality risk: a meta-analytic review." *PLoS Medicine* 7, no. 7 (2010): e1000316.
http://www.plosmedicine.org/article/info%3Adoi%2F10.1371%2Fjournal. pmed.1000316

2. Friedman, Howard. *The Longevity Project: Surprising Discoveries for Health and Long Life from the Landmark Eight Decade Study*. Hay House, Inc., 2011.
http://library.wur.nl/WebQuery/clc/1963174

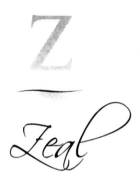

Zeal

"*My mission in life is not merely to survive, but to thrive; and to do so with some passion, some compassion, some humor, and some style.*"

—Maya Angelou

Zeal is a synonym for passion. I think it's a fitting note to end on.—Living a life of passion, and leaving a legacy.

I tell my kids that I hope they find what really inspires them in life. I tell them they are lucky if they can figure out what motivates them, and hopefully they are good at it. I tell them they are even luckier if they can get paid for it! I feel blessed that my life's work is something that I feel passionate about—helping people reach their optimal health and empowering people to have a high quality of life.

I see legacy as leaving something behind that's meaningful; contributing something that you believe in, something that you're proud of, something that will have a positive impact on others that is genuine and lasting. The legacy I want to leave behind is for people to know that I loved them, that I did my best to take care of them; that I cared about people in general, and them in particular. That I always wanted to be better, that I always wanted to learn, and I always wanted my learning to contribute to the benefit of others.

I want to make the world a better place by helping the people I treat feel better so they can live more meaningful lives. I want to help them to be a better version of themselves. I always tell my patients, "I want you to be the best version of Cathy," or Maria, or Steve. I am constantly trying to be the best version of myself as well, and I realize that's a work in progress. It's not a goal that you *reach*; it's a goal that you *live*.

One of the things I am passionate about in my work is cosmetic medicine. It allows me to be creative and practice the "art" of medicine. I tell my patients that their face is my canvas. I like the natural look—I want to enhance your beauty, not cover it up. Because of my training as a family doctor, I am used to looking at and taking care of the "whole" patient. In my work, I initially like to focus on health because my philosophy is "health is beauty." My goal for my patient is to be healthy from the inside out. If I can balance my patients' hormones, their skin is always better. Many times our skin is the outward manifestation of how healthy we are inside. It is my experience that once people feel better on the inside, they want the outside to match. It is so much fun for me to use my skill and artistic eye to slow down the aging process, and I do it with zeal!

Earlier in the book we talked about *com*passion, and I feel that you can't have *compassion* unless you have *passion*. I want to live my life with compassion, which means with love. My passion is for people; my passion is to help others be the best that they can be. I want to empower people to take control of their health, to know that they have options that are not harmful to them, to be confident that they can live a meaningful life.

I know I am a better doctor because I am passionate. I often see people in my profession get burnt out, and there's a lot of research and discussion about how to prevent burnout among physicians.[1] It's a stressful job. My days are long, and can be very tough. I start my day taking care of my family, dropping kids off at school, and then I have a long day at work. Many days I work through lunch. I have patients booked four to five weeks in advance, and people depend on me. People from all over the world come to see me, because they know I care about them. I was impressed when a gentleman came from Switzerland to see me for testosterone pellets. He said that his brother came to see me and I changed his life. He wanted to be like his big brother. I feel privileged to take care of my patients and privileged that they trust me—and I think that's because they know that I'm sincere in my concern for them, and I do my best to be the best doctor I can be!

Integrative and functional medicine has many advances and is cutting-edge medicine. Because I want to learn as much as possible and continue to be better, I go to conferences regularly. I continue to read and I keep abreast of the latest trends. That comes from a passion to be the best, to always learn more, so I can help people reach optimal health. If I didn't have that passion, I don't know if I could get through the day smiling. I can truly say at the end of the day that I feel good about my day's work. I can work a 12-hour day and at the end still have zeal and energy for my family, because I'm doing something that I love to do!

I have a passion for quality of life. My focus on healthy aging is rooted in that passion. I left mainstream medicine and entered this field initially as a result of my own quest to have optimal health, and once I succeeded at that, I wanted to share what I had learned with others. Some of the ways I have done that are through speaking at the community level as well as talking individually with prospective patients about their health choices. I have also had the wonderful opportunity of being a medical contributor for San Diego Fox 5 News. I am honored to have a platform to discuss relevant health topics and share my passion of health with my audience.

My favorite part of Fox 5 News is the "Ask the Moms" segment, which I've been doing for the last two years. "Ask the Moms" is a weekly segment on our local morning news show on Fox 5 featuring three moms—myself, a clinical psychologist, and a blogger—and we talk about relevant parenting topics, with questions from real parents asking for advice on child rearing and health issues. I am so grateful to Leslie Marcus, the genius behind "Ask the Moms" and so many other creative segments during her tenure at Fox 5. I appreciate that she believed in me and has been a continual source of motivation through her extraordinary talent and work ethic. I love being part of this show, because one of the things I'm most passionate about is being a good mother. I knew from the time I became a mother that it was going to be the most important job that I could ever have. I am excited to share the experiences I've learned from raising my four kids. My kids make me a better person!

Getting this book out is important to me because it's a part of fulfilling my passion of educating people about the fact that they have choices regarding their health. I really want to share the knowledge I have gained regarding integrative and anti-aging medicine, because I know that there are so many people who don't realize they have options. I want people to know that they can take care of their health in a way that isn't harmful, and many times without prescription drugs. Sometimes you need prescription drugs, and because I am a medical doctor, I bridge the two worlds of functional and mainstream medicine. I know that many people are drawn to me and my clinic because I am passionate about what I do.

I love the quote from Mark Twain, "The two most important days in your life are the day you were born and the day you find out why." Most of us spend at least part of our life searching to find out why we are here, and when you figure out why you are here, it's usually in connection with something you're passionate about. When you discover what you're passionate about, it makes your life so much more meaningful. It helps you to feel more fulfilled in the work that you do and the life that you lead. I think it's so important to stay true to that passion.

I started this book with a chapter on being authentic, and now I'm concluding by talking about living an authentic life—to me, living with passion *is* being authentic. We've talked about many aspects of being authentic. We've looked at how our lives can be more meaningful with good relationships, friendships, hobbies, regular exercise, and eating right. Every one of those things is better with passion!

The most fulfilling or gratifying things I have done in life, I did because they were a true calling for me or I felt passionate about them—or both. And things I wasn't good at, or failed at, were things I didn't have passion for. There are certain guiding principles I follow. I want to always do the right thing. I always want to be kind, respectful, and make sure that people I love know that I love them.

I'll conclude with a quotation attributed to Howard Thurman: "Don't ask yourself what the world needs, ask yourself what makes you come alive and then go and do that. Because what the world needs is people who have come alive." I really believe that the best thing you can do for the world is to do what you are passionate about. Be true to it, pursue it, and you will leave a legacy that you can be proud of.

ACTION:

VISUALIZE YOUR LEGACY

Imagine that you've come to the end of your life. How do you want to be remembered?

What do you want people to think about when they think of you? Journal about what comes to mind.

NOTES:

1. Swetz, Keith M., Sarah E. Harrington, Robin K. Matsuyama, Tait D. Shanafelt, and Laurie J. Lyckholm. "Strategies for avoiding burnout in hospice and palliative medicine: peer advice for physicians on achieving longevity and fulfillment." *Journal of Palliative Medicine* 12, no. 9 (2009): 773–777. **http://online.liebertpub.com/doi/abs/10.1089/jpm.2009.0050**

RESOURCES

Dr. Melinda Silva's office is in San Diego and can be contacted in the following ways:

Phone: 619-761-1574

Email: staff@drmelindasilva.com

Address:

890 Eastlake Parkway, Suite 305

Chula Vista, CA, 91914

Don't miss out on our monthly newsletter that highlights latest medical trends and features clinic specials. Please visit my website at www.drmelindasilva.com and enter your email. We respect your privacy and do not share your email.

To find out more about Age Defense Water (discussed in Trust Yourself) or to order it in bulk, go to www.agedefensewater.com

To order mineral makeup or Cardio to Go supplements, please visit my website at www.drmelindasilva.com and click on Youngevity makeup and supplements.

ABOUT THE AUTHOR

Melinda Silva, MD, is a Board-Certified physician and uses her expertise and training to provide the best medical care to her patients, with a focus on prevention and holistic healthcare. The goal of her compassion-centered practice is to blend allopathic medicine with complementary medicine, bridging the two disciplines.

After 16 years as a Family Doctor and after treating her own perimenopausal symptoms with alternative therapies, Dr. Silva opened her own Anti-Aging practice with an emphasis on optimal health with body, mind, and spiritual rejuvenation. Her professional goal is to improve the quality of life of others by focusing on the root cause of disease instead of just treating symptoms. She has helped to train other doctors in her field, lectured at a national level, has been featured on CBS' "The Doctors," and serves as a medical contributor for Fox 5 News.

Dr. Silva specializes in bioidentical hormone therapies, weight loss, and cosmetic medicine. She is able to use hormones to help people with weight gain, hair loss, chronic pain, insomnia, fatigue, stress, lack of energy, low libido, and mood changes. Dr. Silva acknowledges that lifestyle factors including nutrition, sleep, and exercise are crucial for a healthy mind and body. Dr. Silva has received numerous awards and accolades for quality clinical care, academic excellence, teaching, leadership achievement, and philanthropic service. She is most honored by a Compassionate Care award nominated by her patients.

Dr. Melinda Silva has dedicated most of her life to community service. She has volunteered to help abused and neglected children, tutored teens in juvenile prison, provided free medical care to the homeless, and organized an outreach program to mentor high school students. From soccer mom to Girl Scout troop leader, Dr. Silva is enthusiastic to be a role model and make a positive impact on those around her. Dr. Silva lives in San Diego, California, and is inspired most by her husband Rafael and their four children, Rafi, Danny, Christian, and Aliana, who give her endless joy and remind her of what is most important in life.

CPSIA information can be obtained at www.ICGtesting.com
Printed in the USA
LVOW10s1410200115

423600LV00017B/289/P